"When Irma Rombauer published *The* [...] imagined we'd need to learn to eat with joy eighty years later. But we do. Stone offers the backstory of our current food woes and dilemmas along with hopeful and redemptive responses. And all the while she invites us toward a practical, joyful celebration of just, good food."

LISA GRAHAM MCMINN, author of *Walking Gently on the Earth* and *Dirt and the Good Life*

"*Eat with Joy* is a perfect title for this wide-ranging look at food and eating. I loved Stone's emphasis on communal meals and finding pleasure in the sensory experience of eating. My creativity—and appetite!—were stimulated by her stories about God's joyful presence in the growing, cooking and savoring of food, and the connections she made between food and justice were illuminating. The variety of beautiful table prayers at the end of each chapter reflect the heart of the book, encouraging the reader to see food as a gift from God to be enjoyed in God's presence and with the people we love."

LYNNE M. BAAB, author of *Fasting, Sabbath Keeping* and *Joy Together: Spiritual Practices for your Congregation*

"In the quest to deal at length in writing with a theology of the ordinary (work, rest, play, study, worship, sex) it turns out I left out a crucial subject—eating. Thankfully Rachel Marie Stone's splendid new book fills the void—in my stomach, mind and heart—for an adequate and accurate theology of eating from a biblical point of view. I'm tempted to give the advice God gave Ezekiel—'eat this book.'"

DR. BEN WITHERINGTON III, Amos Professor of NT for Doctoral Studies, Asbury Theological Seminary

"In this food-focused age, reading about food can be a lot like eating it: fraught with anxiety, confusion, excess and even emptiness. Rachel Marie Stone is here to restore what God intended from the first—real joy. You'll find much wisdom and celebration in its pages, including recipes and simple family-tested ways of living and eating more joyfully right now. Make ready the feast!"

LESLIE LEYLAND FIELDS, editor of *The Spirit of Food*

"*Eat with Joy* is delicious! Generous, wise, well-reported and—yes—joyful, Rachel Marie Stone's book will open your hands so that you may receive the good gifts of God. She had me long before even mentioning saag paneer, *Babette's Feast* or the recipe for cinnamon rolls."

JENNIFER GRANT, author of *Love You More and MOMumental*

"I'm not proud of this, but I didn't start taking my eating habits seriously—or seeing them as part of my spiritual life—until I reached midlife. I wish I'd started when I was in my twenties (or before), and I wish I'd had *Eat with Joy* as my guide. The beautiful mealtime prayers alone are worth the price of the book. A treasure for soul and body."

BRIAN D. MCLAREN, author, speaker, blogger (brianmclaren.net)

"This book is manna in the wilderness to any Christian who has ever had a conflicted relationship with food, thereby missing the unadulterated joy of eating. In a fresh and engaging voice, Rachel Marie Stone reminds us that when we savor delicious, nourishing food, we are actually tasting God."

JANA RIESS, author of *Flunking Sainthood: A Year of Breaking the Sabbath, Forgetting to Pray, and Still Loving My Neighbor*

"In our multitasking, 24/7 world, many of us treat food as mere fuel for our bodies. By slowing down, eating healthier and learning to relish our food, we catch a glimpse of life as God intended: an everlasting communion with him. Those who seek an improved relationship with their daily bread will rejoice in *Eat with Joy*. Highly recommended!"

NANCY SLEETH, author of *Almost Amish: One Woman's Quest for a Slower, Simpler, More Sustainable Life*

"Rachel Marie Stone is a woman after my own heart: a mom, a writer and a Christian who loves to feed the people she cares about. *Eat with Joy* is practical and inspiring, wise and full of love."

SHAUNA NIEQUIST, author of *Cold Tangerines, Bittersweet* and *Bread and Wine: Finding Community Around the Table*, www.shaunaniequist.com

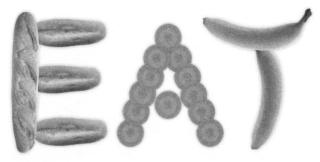

REDEEMING GOD'S

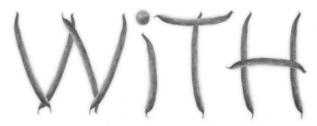

GIFT OF FOOD

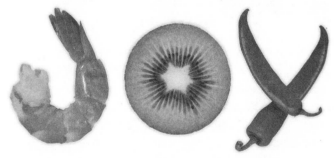

Rachel Marie Stone

Foreword by **Norman Wirzba**

IVP Books

An imprint of InterVarsity Press
Downers Grove, Illinois

InterVarsity Press
P.O. Box 1400, Downers Grove, IL 60515-1426
World Wide Web: www.ivpress.com
E-mail: email@ivpress.com

InterVarsity Press® is the book-publishing division of InterVarsity Christian Fellowship/USA®, a movement of students and faculty active on campus at hundreds of universities, colleges and schools of nursing in the United States of America, and a member movement of the International Fellowship of Evangelical Students. For information about local and regional activities, write Public Relations Dept., InterVarsity Christian Fellowship/USA, 6400 Schroeder Rd., P.O. Box 7895, Madison, WI 53707-7895, or visit the IVCF website at <www.intervarsity.org>.

Scripture quotations, unless otherwise noted, are from the New Revised Standard Version of the Bible, copyright 1989 by the Division of Christian Education of the National Council of the Churches of Christ in the USA. Used by permission. All rights reserved.

While all stories in this book are true, some names and identifying information in this book have been changed to protect the privacy of the individuals involved.

Cover design: Cindy Kiple
Interior design: Cindy Kiple
Images: Red chili peppers: © Svetlana Kuznetsova/iStockphoto
Ripe banana: © Nikolai Klõga/iStockphoto
Green peas: © kyoshino/iStockphoto
Green bean: © John Gollop/iStockphoto
Bread roll: © John Gollop/iStockphoto
Kiwi slice: © Dimitris Stephanides/iStockphoto
Carrot slice: © Dimitris Stephanides/iStockphoto
Baguette: © Cristian Baitg/iStockphoto
Shrimp: © aroax/iStockphoto
Cutlery: © malerapaso/iStockphoto
Measuring cups: © Christopher Conrad/iStockphoto

ISBN 978-0-8308-3658-1

Printed in the United States of America ∞

Library of Congress Cataloging-in-Publication Data

Stone, Rachel Marie, 1981-
Eat with joy : redeeming God's gift of food / Rachel Marie Stone.
p. cm.
Includes bibliographical references and index.
ISBN 978-0-8308-3658-1 (pbk. : alk. paper)
1. Food—Religious aspects—Christianity. 2. Food habits—Religious aspects—Christianity. I. Title.
BR115.N87S76 2013
248.4'6—dc23
2012041420

| P | 18 | 17 | 16 | 15 | 14 | 13 | 12 | 11 | 10 | 9 | 8 | 7 | 6 | 5 | 4 | 3 | 2 | 1 |
| Y | 27 | 26 | 25 | 24 | 23 | 22 | 21 | 20 | 19 | 18 | 17 | 16 | 15 | 14 | 13 | | | |

For my parents,
who fed me good food and good books,
both with great love.

For my children,
who feed me, heart and soul and mind,
with their hunger and thirst for life.

And for Tim, without whom . . .

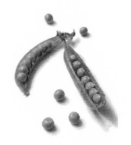

Contents

Foreword by Norman Wirzba 9

INTRODUCTION: CONFLICTED EATING 11
Our Complicated Relationship with Food

1 JOYFUL EATING 23
God's Intent for How We Relate to Food

2 GENEROUS EATING 43
Serving the Needy, Loving Our Neighbors

3 COMMUNAL EATING 66
How Meals Bring Us Together

4 RESTORATIVE EATING 88
How Eating Together Heals

5 SUSTAINABLE EATING 106
Wise Choices in Stewarding the Land

6 CREATIVE EATING 132
Food Preparation as Culture Making

7 REDEMPTIVE EATING 157
Putting Best Practices Together in the Real World

For Further Reading 177

Group Discussion Guide 180

Acknowledgments 187

Notes 189

Name and Subject Index 203

Recipe Index 206

Scripture Index 206

About the Author 207

Foreword

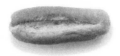

It is hard to imagine an important human event that does not involve eating. Birthdays, weddings, major accomplishments and funerals require eating because the sharing of food is the sharing of life with each other. Today's industrial culture tempts us to think that food is simply fuel or a commodity we need to keep us going through our schedules. But our own experience and desire teach us that is not right. Deep down we know that food is fellowship. When we eat together we share so much more than calories or grams of fat. We share in each other's joy, pain, struggle and hope. Sharing food we share ourselves. We show ourselves willing to be companions in life's journey, people who by sharing bread (*panis*) also share love.

It is no accident, then, that Scripture has food and eating constantly in view. God creates life by creating food. Indeed, among God's most primordial blessings is the grace of food and the promise that agricultural cycles will yield their fruit in due season. God then invites the whole of humanity to participate in the just and generous sharing of food, making hospitality to others a basic witness to faithfulness. God wants us to share food with each other because in doing that we share God's love.

Jesus mirrors the Father in feeding the world. He celebrates the gifts of life together by providing for and eating with everyone, even the outcast and those on the margins of society. Eating together matters because it breaks down the walls of suspicion and hostility that separate us from each other. We should never forget that Jesus was called a glutton and a drunkard (Lk 7:34; Mt 11:19), a sure sign that he understood the importance of a welcoming and festive meal. And then best of all, Jesus institutes a meal—the Lord's Supper—as the regular occasion in which his followers learn to be his continuing hospitable and nurturing presence in the world.

Christian faith and life have always been deeply and inextricably bound up with eating. But Christians have not always appreciated this. What a joy, then, to have the gift of this book by Rachel Marie Stone. In prose that is inviting, nonjudgmental and inspiring, Stone shows us that we can eat with joy, and in such eating extend God's love in the world. By combining stories, recipes, biblically based reflection and numerous practical tips, Stone helps us move more deeply into the mystery and the grace that eating is. Prepare to receive a blessing.

Norman Wirzba
Research Professor of Theology, Ecology and Rural Life
Duke Divinity School
Author of *Food and Faith*

Introduction

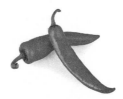

I had gone to the doctor for a checkup before heading to camp, thrilled finally to be old enough to spend twelve hours a day opening giant cans of ketchup to fill dozens of red plastic squeeze bottles, preparing gallons of Jell-O and pouring exactly eight ounces of milk into hundreds of hard plastic cups, all for the love of Jesus and of the hundreds of inner-city children who came to us all through July and August. At fifteen, I'd begun that burst of growth that was changing my stick-thin child's body into a curvier, more "womanly" one. For the first time the doctor's scale registered a number higher than 100. I was proud—*that sounded like a grown-up weight!* And then I moved on to dreaming of the friendships that would be formed and strengthened through the long hours dishing up canned pears in dozens of perfect half-cup portions. Through our welcoming them in Jesus' name, many children who were previously unacquainted with the tradition of three daily meals would be blessed.

It turned out to be a difficult summer.

I met a surfer dude who was into health food and nutritional supplements, who criticized the diet of my beautiful, curvy best friend even as he surreptitiously snapped pictures of her at the pool and who complained that camp food didn't have enough living enzymes or something; I felt guilty when he watched, horrified, as I ate *two* chocolate cupcakes with vanilla frosting. I held hands with a boy who shared his organic fruit spritzer, rolled his eyes at my love of Burger King chicken sandwiches and told me about his family's natural food co-op—something exotic I'd never heard of—back in Park Slope, Brooklyn. I got in trouble for staying out too late one night (*"We expect better from the pastor's daughter!"*), was rebuked for reporting on a mild incident of sexual harassment I'd witnessed and was criticized because the boy whose hand I held was African American, and I was not.

A heaviness came to my abdomen that felt quite literal, as if my anxieties were gathering into a lump in the area of my appendix that grew with each day and especially with each meal. I felt the pounds I'd gained were bad, that *I* was bad, that the hand-holding was too soon (it was, after all, the era of "kissing dating goodbye"), that the way I ate was all wrong—and that somehow these things were connected. The final result was that I no longer felt pride in my "grown-up weight." Instead, as often happens, I felt desperate to dial the number on the scale back to where it had been before life felt complicated.

For ten years following, I struggled daily with an unremarkable eating disorder, which is to say that my story would never make a good *Lifetime* movie, because it was only slightly more dramatic than the eating disorder that most North Americans have: the psychotic notion that we can have it all, eat it all, do a minimum of physical labor and still look both thin to the point of undernourishment and "healthfully" toned and tanned. I absorbed magazines, TV shows and movies uncritically and prescriptively, as if they were saying of the Michelle Pfeiffers and the Cameron Diazes and all the other pretty people: "They're real! Be like them!" When I looked in the mirror, I saw flat feet, thick-ish ankles, undainty kneecaps, broad shoulders, mournful eyes with permanent dark circles and frizzy hair. Everything about my appearance seemed *wrong*. But in America, the possibilities of individual determination are endless—*you can become as rich and as thin as you determine to be!* So I sought to change my body through all the ways that advertisements teach us is possible: the chromium picolinate supplements, the protein shakes, the NordicTrack, the chirpy aerobics videos, the Velcro-fastened ankle weights.

The worst part of the struggle, though, was in my mind.

I hated being obsessed with my body; I hated my body. I was hungry and longed to eat—having always loved cooking and eating food of all flavors and textures, from matzo ball soup to *naan* bread with spicy *saag paneer*—but I was afraid to eat. I wanted to do good in the world, to use gifts I knew God had given me, to read good books and maybe write one someday, but I could hardly get my mind off myself and my jeans' size. The church seemed to have nothing to say that helped. By my lights there was little difference between Christians and non-Christians in attitude toward food, bodies and dieting. I never heard the "make your body perfect" message that screamed from every billboard and TV commercial soundly refuted by some good theology. Instead, while the wider culture was doing Weight Watchers or Jenny Craig, we church people had *Free to Be Thin* and *The Weigh Down Diet*, which baptized the "worldly" desire to be thin for appearance's sake with the dubious motives of discipline and being a "better" (read "thinner") witness for Jesus.

In her book *Seeking the Straight and Narrow*, Lynne Gerber explores two evangelical organizations dedicated to changing bodies as they attempt to change minds and hearts. One is a popular church-based weight loss program; the other aims to help people who are gay become straight. Gerber notes that while people outside evangelical Christianity dispute the ex-gay project, people of all convictions agree on the weight-loss project; even where "God's love for the fat person is affirmed, [it is] modified with a health caveat."[1] When Neva Coyle, author of *Free to Be Thin*, regained weight, she was sharply criticized by her former followers but still managed to see herself as being "loved on a grander scale"—the title of a book that sold poorly compared with books continuing to promise that weight loss and holiness were mutually reinforcing projects. Few, it seems, are open and affirming when it comes to fat. So while the possibility of sexual reorientation is hotly disputed, that of body reshaping is widely and uncritically accepted, even in the face of abundant evidence suggesting that weight loss is rarely achievable or permanent.[2] Nonetheless, the promise of bodily improvement keeps many people locked in a struggle wherein food is the enemy at the gates, the body a city that *could* be glorious if not for the daily necessity of ceding at least some ground to the enemy.

North Americans, on average, spend a smaller percentage of their income on food than any other people on earth now and throughout history, because contemporary industrial agriculture yields an enormous supply of very cheap food. This is in many ways miraculous, and even the most quotidian of our meals are gastronomic wonders if we take a long view of human dietary history. Yet the ordinary wonder of a cheeseburger with lettuce, tomato and fries costing less than ten dollars has created other problems: depleted soils requiring heavy applications of chemicals to yield crops, "dead zones" created by those chemical runoffs, heavy dependence on fossil fuels, mistreated livestock and exploited workers. Additionally, those great surpluses of cheap food—which must be sold somewhere, to someone and, presumably, to be eaten—have helped create the first generation of children with life expectancies shorter than their parents, the result of poor quality food consumed in excessive quantities.

Today, people in the United States spend as much on weight loss products and programs as the federal government spends annually on the Supplemental Nutrition Assistance Program (SNAP, better known as food stamps). The number of people worldwide suffering the ill effects of *too much* food nearly equals the number of people suffering the ill effects of *too little* food; as many are obese to the point of illness as are undernourished to the point of illness. School districts agonize over spending a whole extra quarter per day per child for better school lunches in the same week as the Justice Department releases a financial report showing that they'd paid more for muffins at a single catered event than a family of four receives from SNAP for *six months'* worth of groceries.

The first lady of the United States, Michelle Obama, has launched a "war" on childhood obesity, while the Internet news alerts scream about children as young as four being diagnosed with anorexia. More than one friend tells me of young daughters scared to eat birthday cake because public service announcements have made healthy eating all but a moral imperative. Celebrities swear off the supposedly bloat-inducing gluten (and therefore most grains) while bags of surplus grain are the only thing standing between millions of Somalis and death by starvation. Thousands of North Americans turn up their noses at any food that's not local and/or organic, while thousands more are happy to eat whatever is handed to them at the food pantry or purchased on a shoestring from the local scratch-and-dent. Thousands of others don't give much thought to what they're eating one way or another because they're too busy or too old or too young, or whatever.

People seem to be growing more aware that what we choose to eat, and how, and with whom, has effects reaching beyond our own health, weight and waistlines. Blogs and news sources repeatedly tell us that our sugar, our chocolate and even our *lettuce* sometimes comes to us through the labor of people who are enslaved, either literally or through unjustly low wages—a concern quite apart from the question of whether those foods are "healthy" or "unhealthy." Hardly a week goes by without some undercover video or report documenting the shameful state of what used to be called animal husbandry. At the same time, remarkably self-centered approaches to diet continue apace. I read about an elite New York City "coach" who promulgates a popular approach to weight loss involving exhaustive self-inventories aimed at discovering which foods "work" or "don't work" with each person's body. Clients keep a diary of every single thing they eat and how it makes them feel.[3] I hate to imagine a dozen or so of her devotees trying to plan a dinner party.

But for all the madness, there is more and more talk about a movement, a revolution starting where most revolutions do: with ordinary people. People who love good food and care about the health of the planet—and that of people and animals too—are rediscovering the pleasures of eating and enjoying meals composed of responsibly procured foods, including food that is nostalgically referred to as *heritage*—and helping others enjoy them too. They are rediscovering traditional tasks like vegetable gardening and home preserving. Celebrity chefs as different as Jamie Oliver and Alice Waters have used their fame to help school-age children learn about food, gardening and cooking.[4] Writers like Michael Pollan, Mark Bittman and Barbara Kingsolver have offered compelling and highly personal accounts of their separate quests to find better ways to eat, ways to bring healing to people and the planet, ways to highlight pleasure while preserving health in the fullest sense.[5]

In many important ways, this movement is not new. Awareness of the ecological implications of industrial-scale food production was a part of the environmental movement from the very beginning. A sense that personal consumption might somehow affect others a world away has been with us for even longer. Posters from World War I urged American housewives to "can the Kaiser"—to do their "bit" for the war effort by growing and canning their own food, thereby freeing up American resources for munitions-building. During World War II, Victory gardens and modest rationing were similarly oriented, even where partially symbolic, an attempt to forge national solidarity. In the 1970s, Francis Moore Lappe's *Diet for a Small Planet* and the Mennonite Central Committee's *More-with-Less Cookbook* explicitly connected North American overconsumption with food shortages elsewhere; their recipes and suggestions aimed at changes that were as much philosophical (and, in the case of *More-with-Less*, theological) as practical.[6]

A nation of immigrants, a former British colony in the "New World," the United States has no uniform food culture. Our cuisine has developed from the fertile and fraught exchanges between the land, the people who first lived here and those who have come from elsewhere, reflecting our nation's marvelous diversity and richness as well as our weaknesses and prejudices. We might enjoy Pakistani food for lunch and Colombian cuisine for dinner, overeat steak but turn up our noses at organ meats, forbid children their birthday cupcakes but serve them breakfast cereal consisting of 25 percent sugar by weight. The processed foods appearing on many tables—often loaded with sugar, salt and creatively engineered corn—have left their mark not only on our blood panels but on people's lives a world away. "American food" (as it's referred to elsewhere) is food that's bad for you, and you can get it anywhere. Places that don't have clean water have Coca-Cola. Even countries whose foodways are celebrated—like Italy and France—have seen fast food's effects on the bodies of their people and in their most cherished public spaces. The fact that every few years seems to see the publication of a new guide for Americans to eat more like the French or Italians or another people group may be evidence of the anxiety of this influence.[7]

I was raised in the church—a pastor's daughter no less!—a Christian from the cradle and the kind of girl who would work

hard all summer for pennies for the sake of Jesus and the least of
these (and, to be honest, for the meager glory—not least, the ad-
miration of cute youth group boys—accruing to one willing to do
such a thing). I also had a great trust in the Bible. I suspected the
Bible might somehow assuage, or at least address, my anxieties
about food and my body. In some ways, I pursued my under-
graduate degree in biblical studies to try to fix whatever it was
that was broken in me with respect to food and my body. Though
I'd read the Bible all my life, it remained to me a strange book filled
with odd pronouncements and prohibitions: *Don't mix two kinds of
cloth? God, please knock out my enemy's teeth? Kill all the Canaanites?*

The Bible was also seemingly obsessed with food and, given my
conflicted feelings, even soothingly hospitable passages like the
following filled me with confusion:

> Ho, everyone who thirsts,
>   come to the waters;
> and you that have no money,
>   come, buy and eat!
> Come, buy wine and milk
>   without money and without price.
> Why do you spend your money for that which is not bread,
>   and your labor for that which does not satisfy?
> Listen carefully to me, and eat what is good,
>   and delight yourselves in rich food. (Is 55:1-2)

God seemed to like food and, if anything, to think that a little
fatness was a good thing. People called Jesus a glutton and a
drunkard, a reputation he certainly didn't get by following the
vegan *Hallelujah Diet,* which doesn't allow alcohol or even, mercy
on us, coffee. But was I "gluttonous" for wanting more than bare-
bones survival rations? If I ate for pleasure, wasn't that a sin, at
least according to Augustine and Gregory of Nyssa and other wise
men of the early church? And what of the fact that "holy" people

in history and literature seemed always to be thin, like Mlle. Baptistine Myriel, the sister of the bishop of Digne in *Les Misérables,* whose holiness and thinness were almost indistinguishable:

> What had been thinness in her youth had become in maturity transparency, and this etherealness permitted gleams of the angel within. Her form was shadow-like, hardly enough body to convey the thought of sex—a little earth containing a spark . . . a pretext for a soul to remain on earth.[8]

How could I fuss about learning to bake the perfect chewy brownie when I had hungry neighbors across the street and around the globe? Surely *that* was a pursuit guaranteed never to elevate (attenuate?) me to near-transparent angel status.

But there remains that food and drink appear at crucial points in Scripture, from forbidden fruit to the marriage supper of the Lamb, and dozens of places in between. It's in there more than angels, sexual ethics and heaven, and it's a site of sin, grace, mercy, communion, life and *joy*. At the same time, I tried to figure out what everyone—farmers and poets, chefs and priests, scientists, novelists, mothers and filmmakers—thought about food, how it figured into the landscapes of human lives and imaginations across cultures and throughout history. Sometime during all that reading and writing (and cooking and eating food, and conceiving and birthing children) my fears and conflicts about food and my body changed shape, making room for other ideas and concerns and, more importantly, for other people. After a time and for brief moments, I found that I was able to take greater and greater joy in the Creator's good gift of food.

This book takes its title from Ecclesiastes, a book that laments the futility and brevity of life, a book that reflects (or is reflected in) a good many people's experiences of life under the sun—you work hard and the promotion goes to one less deserving; in all the places and situations you expect justice, you find injustice; the more you

know, the sadder you grow; and no matter how rich or wise or beautiful, we all get old and feeble and die. Turns out the best we can do
is to fear God, love our neighbor and enjoy the good things of this
life with an enjoyment that's tempered by the knowledge that life is
fleeting and that we have obligations to God and to one another.
Nonetheless, the Preacher tells us to eat our bread with joy and
drink our wine with merry hearts; God approves.

What follows are things I've explored on my journey in learning
to eat as a Christian. I'll be looking at biblical perspectives on food
and eating and how they might relate to the insights of those who
have helped build and influence the contemporary food movement,
those who have worked and studied as nutritionists and counselors
and farmers, and those who continue to grow and prepare food in
ways that elevate it to the status of art. These are paths I've explored because of asking questions like, "Which peanut butter
should I buy?" "Which oil did I hear was healthy?" "How come my
biceps don't look like that?" "How do I know what vegetables are in
season, and does it matter?" "Why can't I stop thinking about my
cellulite when two thousand kids died of malaria today?"—things
I've wondered about while at the same time needing to feed my
kids and get on with my life. It's what I've explored on my journey
toward *joyful eating*: eating that is, at its best, joyful, generous, creative, communal, restorative and redemptive, and aimed always at
experiencing more of God's goodness, beauty and grace while
strengthening the ties that bind us to one another and to creation.

In chapter one, "Joyful Eating," I'll talk about how God's provision of food is always a gift to be received with open, grateful
hands. From the Garden of Eden to the Bread of Life, food is a
living metaphor for God's sustaining love for his people, meant to
be accepted with joy.

Chapter two, "Generous Eating," looks at the importance of
serving the "least of these." God demonstrates care and love by
giving food; we're called to be like God by *sharing* food. In the Old

Testament book of Ruth, Boaz goes beyond Deuteronomy's law to share with Ruth, a widow and a foreigner. Though hunger takes a different shape today—U.S. poor are more likely obese than skeletal—Christian obligation to "the least of these" remains unchanged.

In every culture, sharing meals is a powerful sign of acceptance and care. Chapter three, "Communal Eating," looks at the significance of shared meals in Scripture—particularly, at Jesus' meals with "sinners"—and at contemporary evidence that shared meals are essential social "glue," nourishing and uniting people in deeply significant ways. Similarly, chapter four, "Restorative Eating," looks at how eating together is helpful and healing on a number of levels, especially as an effective method for treating eating disorders. These chapters suggest the centrality of the table in the life of Christ's body.

Chapter five, "Sustainable Eating," looks at creation—the natural world that Christians consider God's handiwork. God, who looks at all creation with intimate loving regard, seems especially to delight in biological diversity—the very thing that contemporary agriculture has steadily diminished in response to the alternative values of uniformity, predictability and mechanization: McDonald's needs one specific kind of potato, so that kind—not the thousands of other kinds of potatoes God made—is the kind that's cultivated on a massive scale.

Chapter six, "Creative Eating," looks at cooking and eating as a form of culture making with potential for worship. When we look at elements of food as God does—with loving attention to their peculiar details—and build on the culinary traditions of those who've gone before us, we create a new food culture that builds on old ones while glorifying the Creator in whose image we're created.

The final chapter, "Redemptive Eating," ties together the diverse threads that have run throughout and discusses ways to practice joyful eating in the real world.

You may have had any number of reasons for choosing this book and reading this far. Maybe, like I once did, you struggle with feeling guilty and conflicted about food, your body and with sorting out the confusing messages about them swirling about in our world. Maybe you don't give food too much thought unless and until you're hungry, or maybe the space food takes up in your mind feels intrusive. Perhaps you've been acutely ill with one kind of eating disorder or another. Perhaps justice or ecology or cooking or community living is your passion. Perhaps you're interested in something else entirely.

Whatever your reasons for reading, this book is for you, because you are God's beloved, made in God's own image, and you *eat*. As a fellow traveler in learning to walk with Jesus, to feed on him who is the true Manna and the Bread of Life, I am hoping—even praying—that my words may be a blessing to you; that whatever your story, you may come to eat your bread with ever-increasing *joy*.

1

Joyful Eating

GOD'S INTENT FOR HOW WE RELATE TO FOOD

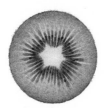

Why do we eat? I remember being a hungry child and thinking a lot about hunger and desire and fullness. Oh, I never felt hungrier than any other North American kid waiting for dinner, but when that empty rumble began in my middle, I'd think of how strange it was that even foods I did not usually prefer began to sound *good*. And how smells that nauseated me when I was full enticed me when I was hungry. And how it felt good finally to begin eating—how quietness would settle my querulous insides as I chewed my bread and butter.

How strange, I thought. *We all have this space inside us that must be filled with food at regular intervals if we're to go on living.* I would watch my parents or grandparents eat and think how strange it was that we all have these *holes* in our faces to put food in. And special places and implements to do all that with: dining rooms, restaurants, tables, plates, silverware. In our family it was impolite, almost taboo, to start putting food in one's mouth without first waiting for everyone to sit down and thanking God for our meal. I'd consider all the work that went into getting

dinner on the table, the long journey of wheat, livestock and tomatoes from farms to, say, spaghetti with meatballs and Par-
mesan cheese—all the people and animals and tractors and
trucks and warehouses and supermarkets! How long and complicated and mysterious was the journey of milk from a cow to a
foil-wrapped Hershey bar! We didn't just graze on dry nutritional pellets the way my long series of pet hamsters and mice
did. Our eating was meaningful and full of dimensions. Being of
Jewish heritage, we celebrated Passover in addition to the once-
monthly Communion at our Baptist church.

Why did God make creatures that must eat? God surely
could have designed us differently, without the need for food,
but we have a world where people—and virtually everything
else, even microscopic bacteria—eat, or at least do something
that's a lot like eating. And we do it in intricate webs of inter-
dependence, where plants feed from soil and sun and organisms
too tiny to see, animals from plants, humans from all, and all
from God.[1]

And why did God make eating so pleasurable? The biological
explanation—food is pleasurable so that we'll eat it, mere in-
centive for survival—is legitimate in its place, but it doesn't go
far enough. It can't account for Le Cordon Bleu and fine wine,
or chocolate for that matter, though some writers have attempted to defend the culinary arts as an extended preliminary
to sexual activity. Biology has its own story; theology, a different one. Surely God could have designed us with some kind
of human photosynthetic process, or created our refueling
mechanisms in a way that would afford about as much pleasure
as I imagine my laptop derives from being plugged into the
electrical outlet. I suspect and prefer to believe that God made
eating sustaining, delicious and pleasurable because God is all
those things and more. When young students begin at *yeshivot*,[2]
they are given a dab of honey on squares of wax paper—and

admonished: *"Never. Forget. What. God. Tastes. Like."*[3]

Scripture describes the Garden of Eden as a place of abundant, beautiful, delicious food. Yes, Adam and Eve are the keepers of the garden, with work to do, but in those early chapters of Genesis, they don't pore over books on orchard-keeping and worry over the blossoms on fragile young trees the way my husband does each spring. Instead they are called into being among trees already laden with ripe fruit, God having fussed over the fine points of pruning and fertilizing beforehand. The garden is picturesque, fragrant and shaded by "every tree pleasant to the sight and good for food" before any person exerts herself, suggesting that perhaps we eat because God, having prepared for and welcomed us as honored guests, loves to feed us.

The image of God is "male and female"—God's trinitarian life is mysteriously hinted at in the one-yet-two-ness of *ha 'adam*[4]— and so not Adam alone nor Eve alone eats; *they* eat, fed by God. But one thing is withheld, and that Withheld Thing—not the abundant Allowed Things—becomes the obsession and focus of the couple, of the serpent and of the story. Dining with the serpent instead of God,[5] Adam and Eve disrupt their idyllic community, fertility and joy, no longer walking naked and trustfully, enjoying peaceful communion and delicious food with God and one another. Getting food becomes burdensome, backbreaking, at least as much drudgery as delight.

God *wants* to feed people. In keeping the one tree from them, God protected Adam and Eve. When they broke table fellowship with God, they suspected that God was withholding something good, that this "good" thing would make them *like God.* Yet indeed they were already like God, participating in and mirroring the loving communion of the Trinity; serving, guarding, loving all that God had made. So in wisdom, God gave them the independence they had already chosen—to go out from the garden and grow their own food.

These questions of dependence, independence and rebellion center around *food*. Adam and Eve's failure breaks fellowship with God, not just by *doing* what God said not to, but by standing God up, by not letting God do what he wanted to do for them—and what God wanted to do was *feed* them.

BREAD FROM HEAVEN

Imagine that your spouse, roommate or whomever you live with does all the food shopping and cooking for your household day in, day out, week after week. And imagine that it's a task she hates, but (for some reason) there are no alternatives. Perhaps you and the other housemates work too late or are unable to cook. She often complains, "Can't someone *else* prepare the food? I'd be happy eating just about anything if only someone else would cook it." Now imagine one day the skies open up, pouring out pancakes, sandwiches and steak dinners—plus cookies and milk—every day, all freshly prepared and ready to eat.[6] You imagine that your household cook will be delighted—no more shopping, no more cooking, just sit down and eat the well-balanced, delicious food that's falling from the sky onto her plate.

But your cook is anything but happy. She's found at least as many reasons to fret as before. The steak is tough; she prefers pulpy orange juice; she'd rather not have such heavy meals in the evening. And even though the meals fall from the sky every day and at predictable times, she can't stop worrying whether breakfast, lunch and dinner will *really* keep on coming. So at mealtime when everyone else is sitting around laughing and talking and enjoying the food, she's running around collecting extra food in Tupperware to stock your already-stuffed fridge against the day she's sure is coming: the day when the food will no longer fall like rain.

The story of the manna in the wilderness is something like that.

I see in the manna story a beautiful suggestion that, for a time, God reverses the curse of Genesis to again feed his people as he did in Eden. Again, all they have to do is reach out and take from what God has already given.

The manna story takes place just after God has done something amazing and impossible: he delivered Israel from Pharaoh's army by making a pathway through the sea. Surely this God can be trusted. Still breathing the sea air, the Israelites begin to form their complaints and to wish themselves back in Egypt, not least for the food: "If only we had died by the hand of the LORD in the land of Egypt, when we sat by the fleshpots and ate our fill of bread; for you have brought us out into this wilderness to kill this whole assembly with hunger" (Ex 16:3).

God has done the unbelievable in their midst and on their behalf, and five minutes later they're accusing God of plotting to commit mass homicide by starvation. "Okay, okay, everyone calm down," God says, promising to "rain bread from heaven" on them. God's setting up a test to see if Israel will trust this time. It's a bit like a faith-fall exercise, where you fall backward into your partner's arms without looking back or trying to catch yourself. Will Israel fall into God's arms without looking back, or will it try to catch itself?

So God rains manna in the mornings, telling the Israelites to gather *just what they need* for each day, except the sixth day, when they're to gather enough for that day plus the Sabbath. Some people try to hoard food on Monday, worrying about what will happen on Tuesday, but Monday's food stinks and is crawling with maggots by then. Others scoff and put their feet up on Friday, thinking there will be more tomorrow. But there isn't. Just like in Eden, it's hard to trust that God isn't going to hold back the good things, the *best* things; that reaching out and taking what God is offering is really the best bet.

BEING FED BY GOD

As Creator, God loves and cares for all his creation, wanting very much to be in loving relationship with us, wanting us to come with open, empty hands to be filled. I suspect we too often think of God as a cosmic killjoy, waiting to catch us at something "bad" so he can spoil our fun. Yet maybe God is more like a loving parent, waiting to welcome us home with a hug and a bite of something to eat.

Several years ago some outrage arose over the cover photo on *Babytalk* magazine, which depicted a nursing baby gazing up at his mother with adoring eyes, cheek and breast meeting in beautiful symmetrical curves. Some readers were astonished (though the photo was, in fact, very discreet); some wrote angry letters to the editor.[7] Others pointed out that perhaps as a culture we've forgotten what breasts are *for*.[8]

When our first son was newborn, my husband took endless photographs of him in all his varied states, but especially he loved photographing us nursing. I remember picking up the prints and gently chiding my husband, "Why are there *so many* pictures of us breastfeeding?" He said simply, "It's beautiful."

Two and a half years later, when we had another son, photographs again captured our baby's first attempts at nursing. Several years later, I'm grateful we have the photos. I still think a mother and baby nursing is a beautiful sight. The bond of love and security between mother and baby is promoted and nurtured in the act of nursing, even on the level of brain chemistry.[9] Giving food and giving love become one as mother and baby unite physically in breastfeeding, an act of great tenderness, overflowing with metaphoric potential.[10]

As in the *Babytalk* outrage, and in the periodic media flare-ups involving mothers being chastised for feeding babies in various public places, nursing's beauty is poorly understood in much of Western culture. Female breasts have been looked at as primarily sexual, rather than live-giving and nourishing. With refreshing honesty, the Bible uses nursing and breasts to talk about God's care for his people:

> Can a woman forget her nursing child,
>   or show no compassion for the child of her womb?
> Even these may forget,
>   yet I will not forget you. (Is 49:15)

> For thus says the LORD:
> "I will extend prosperity to her like a river,
>   and the wealth of the nations like an overflowing
>   stream;
> and you shall nurse and be carried on her arm,
>   and dandled on her knees.
> As a mother comforts her child,
>   so I will comfort you;
> you shall be comforted in Jerusalem." (Is 66:12)

Like infants with their mothers, we're helpless before the God who feeds us, cares for us and embraces us with *even greater devotion* than that of a loving mother with nursing babies.[11] Does a nursing babe have to "be good" to earn that love—to deserve that tender, intimate feeding? No. He has only to open his mouth and be fed.

And so with us.

My friend's baby girl briefly went through a period of refusing to nurse. That infant cried and cried and cried until at last she fell into an exhausted sleep. Finally, in a groggy state, she'd suckle and feed. A mother's body is wired to respond to her baby's cry, and so my friend's body literally ached to satisfy her baby's hunger as she cried on and on, refusing to eat—it *hurts* not to feed a hungry baby! Painful breast engorgement typically follows late miscarriages or stillbirths, the mother's very body grieving the absence of a hungry newborn. I imagine that this is but a picture of God's parental grief when his people reject his goodness:[12]

As an eagle stirs up its nest,
and hovers over its young;
as it spreads its wings, takes them up,
and bears them aloft on its pinions,
the LORD alone guided him;
no foreign god was with him.
He set them atop the heights of the land,
and fed him with produce of the field,
he nursed him with honey from the crags,
with oil from flinty rock. . . .
You were unmindful of the Rock that bore you;
you forgot the God who gave you birth.
(Deut 32:11-13, 18)

Throughout the Bible, it's clear that God desperately loves, cares for and wants to *feed* the people he has created. God plays the role of Jewish grandma, eager to see you eat his cooking. My own great-grandmother, who in her nineties subsisted almost entirely on chocolate, hovered over me and all my cousins like an anxious mother bird: "Have more soup! Have more noodles!" Once, when everyone was diving into lo mein at a Chinese restaurant, someone overheard her say under her breath: "This is so good. I like this, everyone eating." My own mother (a Jewish grandma now herself) watches her grandsons eat waffles or French toast or scrambled eggs with as much satisfaction and pride as if she were watching them play a Rachmaninoff piano concerto, delighted just to see them accept the love—via food— that she offers.

It's hard for us humans to believe that our best good really is in and from the God who made us and loves us so dearly. We're like sheep that keep veering off pasture to clomp along grassless paved roads.

We need a Good Shepherd.

I AM THE TRUE MANNA

Wendell Berry famously quotes the poet William Carlos Williams:

There is nothing to eat
seek it where you will,
but the body of the Lord.
The blessed plants
and the sea, yield it
to the imagination
Intact.[13]

It's much like what Jesus says in John 6, when he declares, "I am the true manna." The Israelites' desert manna sustained their lives in a land that could not. Of course, all the people who feasted on manna were long dead and decayed by Jesus' time. He's promising something different: that everyone who feasts on him will *not* die: "I am the living bread that came down from heaven. Whoever eats of this bread will live forever; and the bread that I will give for the life of the world is my flesh" (Jn 6:51).

It's just a metaphor. Or is it?

Earlier in that same chapter, Jesus takes one boy's little lunch, feeds five thousand people with it and has some left over. After miraculously filling physical bellies with bread and with fish, the people seek him out the next day to learn more; it's *then* that he explains: "Those who eat my flesh and drink my blood have eternal life, and I will raise them up on the last day; for my flesh is true food and my blood is true drink. Those who eat my flesh and drink my blood abide in me, and I in them" (Jn 6:54-56).

We must, Jesus says, become one with him, to trustfully savor his goodness even more than we trust the things that support our physical existence. Yet, mysteriously, those things that support our existence—the bread, the fish—are somehow more than symbols of his love. Our lives on earth come to an end—only the Bread of Heaven sustains us beyond that return to the dust. Even the frequently dull Peter gets it: "'Lord, to whom can we go? You have the words of eternal life. We have come to believe and know that you are the Holy One of God" (Jn 6:68-69). Certain that *his* best good isn't elsewhere, in this moment at least, Peter is not tempted by forbidden fruit or convinced that the best stuff to eat was back in Egypt. He's partaking of the Word Made Flesh—the Bread of Heaven.

I love that Jesus feeds the people with *physical* bread before revealing himself as the Bread of Heaven, just as I love really eating the bread and the wine when celebrating Communion. Jesus didn't say, "*Think* this in remembrance of me," or "*Say* this in remembrance of me." He said that when we eat and drink, we *do* those things in remembrance of him. William Carlos Williams's poem aligns beautifully with the biblical story here, pushing it forward into our own lives—there *is* nothing to eat except "the body of the Lord."

Jesus as Bread of Heaven is spiritual truth but also *living metaphor*. We eat every day—several times, if we are so lucky; without food, we die. We can no more *make* food grow than we can make rain fall. We are, as Wendell Berry writes, "living from mystery," dependent on forces we can't control and processes we can't fully understand. A physical reality—our bodily dependence on food and, in turn, on the sustaining hand of the Creator who designed the earth to bring forth food—daily reminds us of a spiritual reality: our dependence on Christ. Thus every meal is sacramental: a tangible, tasty reminder of Christ's sacrificial love,[14] especially when we take a moment before eating to consider the potato casserole or Pad Thai (or whatever!) as God's sustaining love made edible.[15]

FEEDING ON CHRIST—EVEN UNAWARE

Contemporary celebrations of the Eucharist (or Mass or Communion, depending on your church tradition) don't quite look like those celebrated in the early days of the church. While I love and cherish aspects both of the Anglican Eucharist that is now my own practice and the Baptist Communion that I grew up with, I've always been intrigued to think that the early church shared all their meals in common, that their breaking of bread in remembrance of Christ truly satisfied their physical hunger while also proclaiming Christ's death and resurrection.

In the multiethnic Baptist church I attended as a child, the Chinese congregation cooked and served a simple meal after Sunday services. I think everyone contributed a dollar or so for the meal. Mostly it was the Chinese members who ate, but I was always hungry during the 11:00 a.m. service. As the delicious fragrance of rice and some kind of sauce wafted through the sanctuary during the worship service, I would tug my mom's arm and beg to stay and eat. Though I never considered that we might have been celebrating the Lord's Supper when we ate that delicious food off of planet-destroying Styrofoam in the church basement, hunched over our plates while perched on cold metal folding chairs, I now feel sure we were.

Spoiler Alert If you haven't seen the film* Babette's Feast, *you may want to skip this next section and see the film before coming back!*

The beautiful film *Babette's Feast*, based on the Danish writer Isak Dinesen's short story, tells a story of grace given by means of food to people undeserving and unaware. A French woman, fleeing her country in the midst of its bloody revolution, takes refuge in the home of two spinster sisters on the coast of Jutland. They're the daughters of a dear departed eccentric, the leader of a small ascetic sect that greatly valued the spiritual above the physical, living lives of extreme simplicity, devoted to kindness and service to others. Suspicious of pleasure (baptized in lemon juice, my dad might say), they eat just what they need to survive, speak as few words as possible and renounce their romantic and

artistic inclinations to devote themselves to their father and to
spiritual pursuits.

Babette, destitute but grateful to have escaped alive, can't
speak Danish but comes with a note from a mutual friend—
"Babette can cook." So the sisters give her the task of preparing
the daily meals of bread soaked in beer, dried fish and similarly
bland foods. She does this faithfully, gently and quietly serving
the sisters as well as the sick members of their congregation. Her
only connection with her old life is a French lottery ticket, renewed for her annually by a friend back home. When she wins
10,000 francs—enough for her to move back to France—she
begs the sisters to allow her to serve all the congregants a delicious meal to celebrate what would have been their father-
pastor's one hundredth birthday.

Alarmed by Babette's proposition, and by the exotic ingredients procured from France, including a live tortoise and a cage
full of quail, the sisters and their small church feel certain that
Babette's feast will lead them into sensual indulgence or something unimaginably worse—a "witches' Sabbath" maybe. Yet, as
she has asked nothing and served faithfully all these years, and
as they don't wish to insult their gentle, mysterious friend, they
agree to the banquet but vow to "become as if they had lost their
sense of taste."

Shortly before the meal, an unexpected guest—one sister's
former suitor, now a famous general—joins their party, making
them twelve in number, the same number Jesus served at the Last
Supper. As his tablemates struggle to resist enjoying the extraordinary food and wine Babette serves them, the cultured general
is astonished, recognizing the meal's extreme luxury. Verbally in-
terpreting the meal for the provincial group—*This is a rare vintage
Veuve Cliquot! This is Cailles au Sarcophage!*—he rightly concludes
that this meal, in that place, was nothing short of a miracle, basing
his speech on Psalm 85: "Steadfast love and faithfulness will meet;

righteousness and peace will kiss each other" (Ps 85:11).[16]

As they eat—enjoying the food despite their resolve not to taste it—the elderly congregants enter into a peace in one another's company quite unlike anything they have shared before. They forgive old grudges and reignite flames of romance.

Afterward, the sisters thank Babette, assuming that she'll soon return to Paris with her newfound wealth. Babette reveals the truth: she was once chef of France's finest restaurant, and she is now penniless once again, having spent the entire sum of her lottery winnings on the glorious meal. She has given all she had—materially as well as artistically—to serve people unable, even *unwilling*, to recognize what they had been given. And yet, in eating the feast, they were blessed. Isak Dinesen writes, "Infinite grace . . . had been allotted to them, and they did not even wonder at the fact."[17]

I think we are all those elderly villagers. Christ himself feeds his very body and blood to us, reluctant people resistant to that feast, barely competent to recognize its magnificence; yet we are no less sustained, renewed and strengthened by it. We're like the daughter, who, tasting the minestrone her mother labored over all day, exclaims, "Mom! If you closed your eyes and tasted this, you'd swear it came from a can!" Or the child who cries because the from-scratch mac and cheese doesn't taste like the boxed kind he loves. We're just learning how to taste the goodness of the Bread of Life.

As in the garden, as in the wilderness, as with God's Word, as with the five thousand and as with the disciples, so with us. There's nowhere to go but to Jesus. He *is* the Bread of Eternal Life.

EATING LIKE CHILDREN

God's grace sustains us even when we come to the table kicking and screaming. But it's more joyful to know—however dimly—the pleasures of Christ's table. How much greater was the general's amazement than the villagers', not simply because experience afforded him appreciation for the fine wine and rare delicacies set before him? He alone had come open to the experience without deciding in advance that he would not enjoy what was to come. They came closed down with fear, suspicion—refusing, as best they could, to be blessed. Though *all* were blessed, was not the general's blessing even more precious because of his candid acceptance of Babette's sacrificial gift?

He came with faith like a child's.

The family therapist and dietitian Ellyn Satter tells this story:

> Seventeen-month-old Holly . . . *loved* to eat. When she was put in her highchair, her eyes lit up, her arms and legs fanned, and she made little squeaking noises. While she ate, she moaned—sensuous, heartfelt moans. Enjoyment *oozed* from her very pores. Delighted friends and family gathered around to enjoy the spectacle.
>
> But Holly's mother was *mortified*. She felt that her daughter's passionate response to food was almost, if not downright, obscene. It meant [to her that] Holly was self-indulgent, a glutton . . . and that she would get too fat.[18]

In time, Holly's mother did what many parents do without exactly meaning to: she taught Holly to fear her pleasure, shaming her and controlling her eating. Holly faced years of disorder before seeking treatment.

Holly's mother might have done better to leave her daughter alone. In a 1928 experiment studying the food choices of recently weaned children living in an orphanage, pediatrician Clara Davis found that children allowed to choose freely from a variety of healthy foods ended up selecting a remarkably balanced diet over time. Her research indicates that children are best left to choose for themselves among a preselected variety of healthy foods. Unlike many adults, they're experts at eating when hungry, stopping when full and somehow intuitively meeting their nutritional needs. Adult interference (as well as the druglike effects of junk foods) can interrupt children's God-given ability to self-regulate.[19] Satter's "eating competency" therapy encourages adults to recultivate these attitudes—positivity and curiosity about food, confidence in their ability to choose—in themselves.[20]

Stories like Holly's remind me of Matthew 19, where the children came to be blessed by Jesus only to face rebuke. The disciples had quickly forgotten Jesus' words: "Unless you . . . become like children, you will never enter the kingdom of heaven. Whoever becomes humble like this child is the greatest in the kingdom of heaven" (Mt 18:3-4). As nursing babes go to the breast with gusto, as toddlers dive into finger foods ready to enjoy, so we should feed on the Bread of Life—anticipating pleasure, prepared to accept goodness and ready to give thanks. This is true of our acceptance of Christ spiritually. But our ordinary eating is sacramental too. It's there to teach us how to taste the Bread of Life, if we open ourselves in that way to the feast.

Joyful eating recognizes God as Creator of heaven and earth and of you and me. God has made food for our bodies, and our bodies for food, including all the sensations and associations that make eating pleasurable and satisfying. We should revel in—not be ashamed of!—our enjoyment of the simple pleasures of smelling, tasting and chewing. When we are fed, it is God who feeds us.[21]

I want to be clear at this point that God's intention and design for creation is that *all* should be well fed. In the brokenness of our world, this is not so; there is a broad gap between God's ideal and the reality of hunger in our world, owing in large part to the human resistance to *sharing*. The Old Testament insists on lavish generosity: "Open thine hand wide unto thy brother, to thy poor, and to thy needy, in thy land" (Deut 15:11 KJV). When we eat redemptively—a concept I will explore in detail later—we honor God's desire for all to be fed by taking action to close that gap. This awareness that brokenness, greed and apathy lead to hunger does not diminish the reality of pleasure or the importance of gratitude. It can, however, encourage us toward temperance in our appetites.

In their place, food and an appetite for it are, like the rest of creation, very good. Ideally, we should come to the table mindful of our Creator and filled with thankfulness, ready to receive with joy what is before us—not, as much of our discourse would have it, focused on calories, fat, restriction, "rightness" or shame. This is not to say that eating with joy is a license for gluttony, which is a destructive distortion of true enjoyment, a case of pursuing desire past the point of pleasure—only that fear of becoming gluttonous should not hamper our pleasure in eating. Some of Ellyn Satter's research indicates that, in fact, taking *more*—not less—pleasure in food leads to *less* overindulgence.

The kind of pleasure I'm suggesting can be somewhat countercultural for those living in North America. Psychologist Paul Rozin has demonstrated that North Americans tend to associate food with guilt instead of pleasure. French people might associate "holiday dinner" with happiness; North Americans associate it with overeating. I've heard, "Oh, I shouldn't," and talk of fat and calories and diets between bites of dessert more times than I can count. An alternative might be gratitude for God's good gift of food and an attentive pleasure to all the sensory delights that go along with satisfying our hunger. As Richard Johnson writes: "Joy, like worship itself, is revolutionary, liberating, dangerous and deeply countercultural, enabling us to resist the forces that would seek to enslave us, and to laugh at their absurdities."[22]

And as the old hymn says: *"Hast thou not seen how all thy longings have been granted in what he ordaineth?"* Praise to the

Lord! (And please pass the bread and butter.)

Joyful eating recognizes the sacramentality of all meals: we "do not live by bread alone." In the film *Sleeper,* Woody Allen's character awakes after 200 years of cryogenic sleep surprised to find all his friends are dead. "But they all ate health food!" he protests, playfully jabbing those who would seek eternal life (or seem to) by means of a perfectly healthful diet; "healthy" eating has in many quarters stepped in as the preferred way to talk about dietary righteousness. But, as Anne Lamott says, we're all "terminal on this bus,"[23] no matter how healthful and plentiful our diets—no matter how many "cleanses" we perform and how many raw greens we ingest. Food sustains our physical life—a good and delightful blessing "under the sun"—but cannot be our all-in-all. It retains its goodness only insofar as we do not make it a "first thing."[24] However, our physical dependence on food can daily remind us of our spiritual dependence on Christ, the only Bread that promises life beyond the grave.

Because joyful eating happens within loving relationship, there is no room for fear and shame. Michael Pollan has quipped that we Americans are a "notably unhealthy people obsessed with the *idea* of eating healthfully." Guilt and anxiety are too frequently our dining partners.[25] There are complicated reasons for this, perhaps even some things we *should* feel guilty about, which is why eating's pleasure must be "extensive . . . not dependent on ignorance." But joyful eating starts with an attempt to recognize food, and ourselves, in light of God our Creator and Christ our Bread of Life. Food is a sign of God's love—and there is no room for fear in love, for love casts out fear.

Accept food like a child, then—joyfully, with pleasure and gratitude.

Finally, joyful eating remembers that we're never "alone with God" and food. The woman in the Garden ate with the serpent and with her husband. The Israelites spurred one another on in greed and doubt. And what kind of story would the "loaves and fishes" be without the disciples to fret and the multitudes to share the meal? Food connects us to others—other people and other creatures—in millions of ways, some visible, many hidden.

And food connects us all to God.

PRAYERS BEFORE EATING

1.
We thank you, Lord, for this our food,
For life and health and all things good.
May manna to our souls be given:
The bread of life sent down from heaven.
In the name of Christ, Amen.

2.
Blessed are you, O God,
King of the Universe,
Who brings forth bread from the Earth.
Traditional Jewish Prayer

3.
God is great and God is good,
And we thank God for our food;
By God's hand we must be fed,
Give us, Lord, our daily bread.
Amen.
Traditional Children's Blessing

4.
May this food restore our strength, giving new energy to tired limbs, new thoughts to weary minds. May this drink restore our souls, giving new vision to dry spirits, new warmth to cold hearts. And once refreshed, may we give new pleasure to

You, who gives us everything.
Irish Blessing

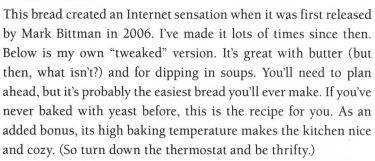

· ·

RECIPES

No-Knead Bread

This bread created an Internet sensation when it was first released by Mark Bittman in 2006. I've made it lots of times since then. Below is my own "tweaked" version. It's great with butter (but then, what isn't?) and for dipping in soups. You'll need to plan ahead, but it's probably the easiest bread you'll ever make. If you've never baked with yeast before, this is the recipe for you. As an added bonus, its high baking temperature makes the kitchen nice and cozy. (So turn down the thermostat and be thrifty.)

In a large glass bowl with a lid, mix together into a loose dough:

3 cups all-purpose or bread flour (up to half of this can be whole wheat; my favorite is Great River Organic flour)
1 1/2 plus 2 tablespoons warm water (about 120° Fahrenheit)
1/4 teaspoon instant yeast
1 1/2 teaspoons salt

Allow this mixture to sit in a warmish place, undisturbed, for 18 hours, until the surface is bubbly. Then, stir down the dough and turn out onto a lightly floured surface. Dust it all over with steel-cut oats, oat or wheat bran, or just some more flour. Allow it to sit for an hour or so longer. Meanwhile, put a heatproof pot or casserole with a lid into the oven and allow it to heat to 450° F. After it has heated for at least 20 minutes, very carefully remove the lid and pot and slide the dough in—it will look messy but end up fine. Cover and bake for 30 minutes undisturbed, then remove lid and finish baking, 10–15 minutes. Turn bread out onto cooling rack and resist the urge to cut into it right away.

. . . .

POINTS FOR ACTION

- Give thanks before each meal and snack. Try to eat slowly and consciously, recognizing the food before you as a sign of God's goodness.

- Read Scripture with an eye toward food and its meaning in the context of the stories and poetry.

- Pay attention to your food with all of your senses. Give yourself a moment to take it in with your eyes, ears, nose and (maybe) hands before you taste, then taste with your full attention.

- Remember that when you eat, you eat in God's presence—always.

- Consider celebrating Communion with freshly baked bread so that it's an extra delight to the senses, and so that your daily bread can deliciously remind you of the Lord's Supper.

2

Generous Eating

SERVING THE NEEDY,
LOVING OUR NEIGHBORS

God feeds our bodies by bringing forth food from the earth in a beautiful living metaphor expressing our ultimate dependence on Christ's loving sustenance. When we share food with people who don't have enough, we do God's work; we do it *for God*. Jesus says as much when he speaks of the final judgment in Matthew's Gospel.

> When the Son of Man comes in his glory, and all the angels with him, then he will sit on the throne of his glory. All the nations will be gathered before him, and he will separate people one from another as a shepherd separates the sheep from the goats, and he will put the sheep at his right hand and the goats at the left. Then the king will say to those at his right hand, "Come, you that are blessed by my Father, in-herit the kingdom prepared for you from the foundation of the world; for I was hungry and you gave me food, I was thirsty and you gave me something to drink." . . . Then the

righteous will answer him, "Lord, when was it that we saw
you hungry and gave you food, or thirsty and gave you something to drink?" . . . "Truly I tell you, just as you did it to one
of the least of these who are members of my family, you did
it to me." (Mt 25:31-40)

When I was in high school, my church youth group fasted and
raised money for World Vision; during the fast, we helped out in
the kitchen of a Coney Island gospel mission. Somehow, I always
thought that feeding people who were hungry—whether a world
away in places of famine or a few neighborhoods away in our own
city—was a cause worthy and good only insofar as it might give us
an "in" to share the gospel verbally. I didn't think that the gospel
was expressed in the making and serving of huge vats of spaghetti
and meatballs, or in going without food to raise money for those
who went chronically without; now I think that the good news—
the gospel—was tangibly, edibly expressed in the shaky hunger of
our fasts and the savory goodness of the food we helped prepare
for hungry people.

I'm not suggesting that feeding the hungry *replace* a verbal declaration of the good news of Christ. But the gospel, as spoken by
Jesus himself, is itself *good news to the poor* and must always be
presented as such. Jesus feeds the multitudes physical bread *before*
telling them that he is the Bread of Life. He heals people's physical
diseases even as he forgives them the sins that disable them from
living as fully as he intends for them to live. A gospel that isn't
good news for people who are poor isn't the gospel. As the apostle
James wrote:

If a brother or sister is naked and lacks daily food, and one
of you says to them, "Go in peace, keep warm and eat your
fill," and yet you do not supply their bodily needs, what is
the good of that? So faith by itself, if it has no works, is dead.
(Jas 2:15-17)

Sharing food was essential to early Christian community life, when believers celebrated the Lord's Supper with a "real" meal that satisfied hunger *while* partaking of, remembering and celebrating Christ's blood and body.[1] Eating and worshiping together *daily*, these Christians held their possessions lightly and opened their hands wide to people who were poor (Acts 2:45). They had understood, truly, what Jesus had said to the rich man: "How hard it will be for those who have wealth to enter the kingdom of God!" (Mk 10:23). Yet though they gave freely, the text tells us that they "ate their food with glad and generous hearts" and that God was blessing them "day by day . . . add[ing] to their number those who were being saved" (Acts 2:46-47). They were being fruitful and multiplying, their words and deeds aligning with the whole goal of God's law, which is, and always was, about loving God and neighbor with a generous, unprejudiced love.

Throughout history, some Christians have taken seriously the command to feed and care for the poor even as others have all but ignored it. Catholic social teaching is a good example of a tradition that takes very seriously Jesus' command to care for "the least of these" as we would care for him. Recently Pope Benedict XVI wrote: "Love for widows and orphans, prisoners, and the sick and needy of every kind, is as essential as the ministry of the sacraments and preaching of the Gospel."[2] On the flip side, Reformed evangelicals Kevin DeYoung and Greg Gilbert have written a book bemoaning the resurgence of enthusiastic evangelical involvement in poverty and hunger relief, insisting that feeding the hungry is, in fact, secondary to the verbal declaration of the gospel:

> It simply **was not** Jesus' driving ambition to heal the sick and meet the needs of the poor, as much as he cared for them. He was sent into the world to save people from condemnation.[3]

My friend Chris, a New Testament scholar and wealth ethicist, points out that Jesus talks more about money than about for-

giveness of sins, heals more people than he pronounces forgiven
and says eternal condemnation is what waits for those who neglect
the poor.[4] And when Jesus, at Judgment Day, separates the sheep
from the goats, he, as Marilynne Robinson notes, "does not mention
religious affiliation or sexual orientation or family values. He says,
'I was hungry, and ye fed me not.'"[5]

There's no excuse for the death of tens of thousands of children
each *day* because they don't have enough food. Feeding the hungry
continues to be a vitally important way to serve Jesus by serving
the "least of these." Still, food justice is a drastically different story
today than it was in Jesus' day. The diseases associated with a
calorie-rich, nutrient-poor diet present at least as serious a global
health crisis. Like malnutrition, poor diet leads to a variety of diseases, like Type 2 diabetes, heart disease and premature death.
Though sometimes referred to as diseases of affluence, especially
when they appear in the global south, these diseases dispropor-
tionately affect poorer people in the US.

In a world in which people are just as likely, if not more so,
to be overfed as to be hungry, is Jesus' concern that people be fed
still relevant?

I believe it is.

THE DISEASE OF GREED

People whose job involves selling junk food or weight loss products
insist that obesity results from a lack of personal discipline,
period. Jillian Michaels bellows on her workout DVDs: "You have
to *fight* for a better body!" The copy on a box of powdered sugar
assures me that an "active lifestyle" (not, apparently, a reduction
in my sugar habit) is the key to good health. Ads on the Internet
and on television promise that their program, their supplement,
their book, their method—*plus your effort!*—will get you thin.
Lobbyists push back against tighter regulations on labeling or
school nutrition standards, insisting, as food companies do, that

"everything in moderation" is fine and that obesity is a question of personal (or, in the case of children, parental) responsibility. What of the millions of children who are extremely obese? Is it really that they lack self-control or parents willing to enforce dietary restrictions, or is it more complicated than that? Maybe Augustus Gloop–worthy greediness is a partial cause of obesity, but I don't believe the situation is nearly as simple as a lack of self-restraint.[6] A hundred years ago, even fifty years ago, Americans had no obesity problem; today, at least a third of Americans are classified as "obese," while another third-plus are "overweight."[7] Did we begin gradually, and then rapidly, to lose self-discipline in the postwar years, especially in the 1970s? Or are other factors in play?

Biologically, we're wired to go wild for salt, sugar and fat—things that are scarce in nature yet energy-rich and necessary for life.[8] Our hard-working hunter-gatherer ancestors knew that if they came upon some wild honey, they should gobble it down; there probably wouldn't be more anytime soon. The taste for sweet things is inborn in humans: breast milk is sweet, and newborns have an intense preference for sweet tastes.[9]

These taste preferences are probably protective mechanisms—a baby's dislike for bitterness means that they're more likely to spit out dangerous or even poisonous plants and substances, and also the pureed veggies we push on them at six months of age. Similar reasons may lie behind the food aversions of pregnant women: the flavors and odors that pregnant women are likely to find repulsive are frequently ones associated with substances potentially toxic to her growing baby.[10]

Foodways are tied to culture: Japanese babies cut their teeth on dried squid, while their French cohorts gnaw the hard end of baguettes, but our pleasure in sweet, salt and fat is inherent to our design. Learning to like the bitterer tastes of vegetables, red wine and dark chocolate is part of growing up, taste-wise.

But the food industry would just as soon keep us all infantile in our cravings,[11] because those primal, inborn cravings are easy and cheap to capitalize on. Many studies demonstrate that children, with their underdeveloped tastes, greatly influence household food-purchasing decisions.[12] Worse, children are not equipped developmentally to critically evaluate advertising or even to distinguish cartoon programming from advertising. When my niece was about five years old, she and I were walking through a store and she spotted a big box of candy with a picture of Shrek on the side. She exclaimed, "Oh, I bet those are good—they have Shrek on them!" I imagined some ad executive rejoicing at her simple faith, wishing fruitlessly that executives cared enough about children's health to limit such endorsements to foods that are actually good for children to eat.[13]

The quintessential fast-food trio of "burger, fries and Coke" perfectly illustrates the food industry's ability to capitalize on our most instinctual taste preferences. Unlike, say, a pot of vegetable stew or a bowl of apple slices, the fast-food trio contains all three potent tastes—salt, sugar and fat in combination—endlessly engineered, tested and retested for "hyperpalatability," making them addictive as well as irresistible. Fast-food chicken tenders—even the kind made with "real" chicken breast—are softened, conditioned, injected, salted, sweetened, coated, fried, tested, retested and adjusted to press all the right buttons in your mouth and brain. As David Kessler explains in *The End of Overeating*, the foods (or, in Pollan's phrase, the "edible food-like substances") dished up by the industry are designed, reworked, tweaked and readjusted to deliver the maximum amount of addictive, "hyperpalatable" effect.[14] This processing tends to increase the number of calories we can eat with minimal effort, much like the effortlessly drinkable "cupcake in a cup" envisioned in the playfully futuristic movie *Wall-E*.

PET imaging shows that on the level of neurochemistry, "hyperpalatable" foods have the same effect on human brains as drugs like heroin, opium and morphine.[15] Tasty, rich food combinations like these were rare and expensive, if not entirely nonexistent, but now they're cheap, ubiquitous and addictive—and food companies know it. Creating irresistible taste and texture combinations and pairing products with packaging and marketing that make you feel good is what food companies stand for. This processing creates much larger profits for their producers than non-processed foods, but in terms of energy value, processed foods are some of the cheapest items in the supermarket. Calculating by cost-per-calorie alone, carrots are four times more expensive than potato chips, and sodas contain some of the cheapest calories in the place.[16]

Which is one reason the people in the United States most likely to be ill with diet-related diseases are also most likely to be the poorest.[17]

The film *Food, Inc.* briefly depicts the story of a Mexican American family who, because of their poverty, are forced to decide between buying vegetables to stay healthy or buying diabetes medications, because they can't afford both. As they visit a fast-food restaurant and a supermarket, the father notes that while a head of broccoli costs $1.69, a chicken sandwich can be had at the drive-through for just $1. Filling up a family of four for $12, in the short run, seems like a very cheap deal. Yet the long-term (and sometimes not so long-term) costs to their health are very, very high.

While places like McDonald's rely on government subsidies—your tax dollars at work!—of corn, soy and other crops to provide the cheap raw materials for processing into burgers, fries and soft drinks, they don't take responsibility for the long-term costs to the health of the poorest and most vulnerable members of American society. It costs a staggering $168.4 billion—16.5 percent of what the US spends nationally on health care—to treat the diseases associated with poor-quality diets.[18] A good portion of that is paid by government programs like Medicaid and Medicare. From beginning to end, the producers and marketers of ever-larger, ever-sweeter, ever-saltier, ever-*present* foods are subsidized by American citizens, while the most vulnerable among us have their quality of life steadily diminished by the consumption of these products. And their companies' shareholders are wealthier for it. Is this food justice for the poor? It takes a different shape than could have been imagined by the biblical authors, but it is certainly no less hated by the same God who declared:

> Hear this, you that trample on the needy,
>   and bring to ruin the poor of the land,
> saying, "When will the new moon be over
>   so that we may sell grain;
> and the sabbath,
>   so that we may offer wheat for sale?
> We will make the ephah small and the shekel great,
>   and practice deceit with false balances,
> buying the poor for silver
>   and the needy for a pair of sandals,
>   and selling the sweepings of the wheat." (Amos 8:4-6)

The poor of today's industrialized countries are less likely to be skeletal, but they're no less at the mercy of corporations practicing deceit with the false balance of "value" meals subsidized by unfair tax benefits and grain subsidies.

I've heard it argued that people have a choice in what they eat and that super-processed foods can be "part" of a "healthy, varied diet," and so forth. Thus, if the poor are more likely to suffer from diet-related disease this must be due to differences in education, exercise habits or something (anything!) besides the fact that the cheapest food is also the least healthy. After all, beans and rice are cheap and healthy, so it must be simply that poor people don't care about good food, a terribly undemocratic and, dare I say, un-American way of looking at things.

Before living for several months as a low-wage worker, Barbara Ehrenreich assumed that she'd be cooking up big vats of lentil soup and other inexpensive foods. The painful truth, as she discovered, is that people who are poor are often more or less forced by their circumstances to buy unhealthy food. Sometimes it's a problem of not having cash up front to pay for the larger, cheaper package of something. Sometimes it's that you need a car to get to a grocery store; if you have to walk, you have to make do with what the mini-mart offers. Plus, if you're living in a weekly-rate motel with no kitchen, that hypothetical pot of lentil stew is nothing more than a nice thought while you tide your hunger over on something from the Wendy's dollar menu.

In *The American Way of Eating*, Tracie McMillan insists that everyone, regardless of income or education level, wants to eat well. But produce is expensive, and urban corner stores—sometimes the only places where people who are poor can shop—are loathe to stock things that can spoil; it's easier to stick to boxes and cans. Yet people who are poor, McMillan discovered, are actually more likely to value produce, especially organic produce; that they purchase less of it is due to its cost. The "reject bins" of produce at the Michigan Walmart where she worked were always empty at the end of the day; apples, she says, went quicker than free donuts. Everyone wants to eat well.

While living in rural California, my husband and I knew some families who lived well below the poverty line. Some of our young friends—teenagers when we knew them—had spent much of their lives sleeping in cars, bathing in the lake and eating things like ramen noodles. For them, "cooking" was stirring up some instant mashed potatoes. When they came to our house for dinner, they brought with them plastic gallon jugs to fill and take home for drinking water. But they didn't mind sampling the vegetable curries and whole-wheat *naan* bread and other "exotic" foods I'd serve. "I've never tasted anything like this, Rachel," said Tony,[19] "but I think I could make it a habit."

If people who are poor in the US are impoverished by the rapacious profit-seeking of food corporations, so, increasingly, are people elsewhere.

A variety of fabulously different eating patterns have kept people healthy and happy for many generations. Inuit people eat lots of blubber to keep warm; Masai people eat largely meat and blood; Pueblo Indians traditionally have eaten corn, beans and squash—diets suited to these people's specific needs and to what their environments provide. Today, an industrialized and globalized food system—a system where just a handful of companies handle everything from farm to processing to plate—threatens traditional foodways everywhere, leading all but inexorably to increased rates of diet-related diseases: high blood pressure, Type 2 diabetes, heart disease and more, even in places with strong food traditions.[20]

The stunning book *Hungry Planet: What the World Eats* shows in large, vivid photographs just how far the super-processed sugary, fatty and salty edibles of the West have made it into the lives of people even in remote corners of the earth.[21] In the film *Babies*, a pair of siblings in remote Mongolia share a bottle of Coca-Cola, that perfect symbol of the globalized, industrialized food system—highly sweet, highly processed, highly advertised and highly packaged product sold the world over. Even places without safe drinking water have Coca-Cola. Even people who have never heard the name of Jesus know the name of Coke.[22]

Is it in any way convincing to suggest that these problems result from a failure of personal discipline? Is Type 2 diabetes the result of gluttony, best fought with prayer and repentance, as Christian diet programs have suggested? Or is the "sin" in our acceptance of this system? If individuals are guilty of lacking self-discipline, corporations are even more so because they knowingly and shamelessly exploit the weaknesses inherent in the human frame for private financial benefit while being subsidized by public funds and blaming the ill effects on the very people they prey upon.[23] This seems to me a clear case of injustice. Does Jesus not also call us to care for those whose lives are diminished by too much bad food—to serve the obese but undernourished poor as well as the starving poor?

STILL A "JUNGLE" OUT THERE

When I was little, my family went out to lunch after church with an older couple—members of the Greatest Generation—and I'd order a hamburger, which I didn't finish. "Rachel, Rachel," Mr. S. chided, "some poor cow gave its life just so that you could have that hamburger. Can't you finish it?" I knew he was teasing me— of course the cow didn't give its life just for my burger. But in my mind's eye, that cow was always standing in a grassy farmyard with a red barn in the background with chickens rooting around nearby for grubs and such.

The documentary *Food, Inc.* introduces Joel Salatin, whose Polyface farm in the Shenandoah Valley looks like that farm I pictured as a child. Convinced that the virtues of accountability and integrity go along with visibility, Salatin built his slaughterhouse as an open-air building. He casually slits chicken throats on film while chatting up his interviewer. Polyface is full of contented animals living much as I believe God designed them to—roaming, scratching and grazing. The people who work there are pretty happy too—having waited two years for a coveted internship, they're doing meaningful work in clean, fresh air.[24]

Contrast this image with the images in the fictional feature film adapted from Eric Schlosser's exposé *Fast Food Nation*. Though the producers of *Food, Inc.* were prohibited by the industry from filming inside real slaughterhouses, *Fast Food Nation*[25] did its best to present a visceral representation of what it's really like inside those places. Simply put, it's a kind of hell, no better (if not worse) than the horrific scenes of injustice, exploitation, danger and abuse described in Upton Sinclair's classic *The Jungle*.

Slaughterhouses are largely staffed by undocumented workers, many of whom are young Latinos. Besides being among the most dangerous jobs in America, they are also one of the most poorly compensated. The mistreatment of animals is upsetting enough, but the human rights abuses that are rampant in the meatpacking industry make me feel like going on a permanent hunger strike. Human Rights Watch released a report claiming that the conditions are so bad as to violate basic human rights.[26]

The 1906 novel *The Jungle* is usually remembered in US history textbooks for leading directly to the rapid passage of the Pure Food and Drug Act and the Federal Meat Inspection Act. Contrary to what I had assumed until I finally read it myself, the book centers not on the gross-out tidbits concerning putrid meat and meat products, but on the life of a meatpacking worker, immigrant Jurgis Rudkus. In the plants Jurgis and his fellow workers face constant speedups, wage cuts and injuries on the production line. They live without decent housing or access to medical care. They are immigrants, fearful of government authorities and unaware of their rights. A hundred years later, they are the same people cutting and packing most of the meat we eat.[27]

For a brief time, from the 1930s to the 1970s, meatpacking jobs were comparable in safety and compensation to other industrial jobs, thanks in large part to worker organizations, which did much to increase the safety of the American industrial workplace, a movement that gathered momentum in the wake of the terrible Triangle Shirtwaist Factory Fire in 1911.[28] But in the 1980s, meat companies began abandoning their multistory urban factories, moving instead to rural areas closer to the confined animal-feeding operations (CAFOs) that supplied the meat. The companies also began to step up the mechanization of the production line, reducing the human jobs to repetitive, mindless cutting—making the same slit on the same spot with the same hand—all day, every day, as fast as possible. At the same time, workers' wages fell drastically. By 2002, wages had fallen by nearly a quarter from what they had been twenty years earlier. The unions were squashed, and undocumented workers made up the backbone of the industry—a population whose vulnerabilities are especially easy for manufacturers to exploit.[29]

Nearly everyone interviewed for *Blood, Sweat, and Fear* "bore physical signs of a serious injury." Occupational Safety and Health Administration (OSHA) reports dryly document some of these gruesome injuries, worthy of a horror movie, which occur at *four times* the rate of illness and injury in private industry:

"Cleaner killed when hog-splitting saw is activated."

"Cleaner dies when he is pulled into a conveyor and crushed."

"Cleaner loses legs when a worker activates a grinder in which he is standing."

Traumatic injuries occur by the thousands in this industry, but even these figures are likely to be artificially low. In the meatpacking plants, accidents are under-reported as a matter of course. Plant managers pressure workers not to report their injuries so as never to be held liable for workers' compensation rights. Yet trauma is only part of the misery: repetitive stress injuries, caused by doing the same motions at high speed thousands of times, also plague many. (I once got a repetitive stress injury in my elbow after *one week* of scooping ice cream.) HRW talked to a man who, though only twenty-two, suffered from "claw hand," his overworked and chronically swollen hands locked in a clawlike position.[30] When workers suffer injuries from slipping on greasy, bloody floors or from working long hours in "cold rooms," company doctors often dismiss their injuries, no matter how severe. One man who tore his Achilles tendon was told by the company nurse, "I don't see any blood, so I can't send you to the doctor."[31]

The novel *Kira-Kira* tells about a Japanese American family working in poultry plants in Georgia, a place that was managed so inhumanely that the workers had to wear sanitary pads to pee into because they didn't get to go to the bathroom often enough. The story is fictional, but the lives it describes are very real.[32] Workers lead lives of miserable poverty while seriously jeopardizing, and in many cases ruining, their health and well-being, and for what? So that chicken breasts can sell at an artificially cheap $2 a pound while Tyson's CEO brings home almost $10 million a year?[33] I'm not saying Jesus is into redistribution per se, but surely he's on the side of reasonable bathroom breaks and wages people can live on. As Tracie McMillan explains in *The American Way of Eating*, food workers' pay is such a small part of food's total cost that worker salaries could be raised substantially with barely perceptible changes to Americans' food budgets.[34]

Marketers are careful to create the impression that our meat comes from places that look like Salatin's Polyface farm, but the reality is far from that. Most of our meat comes from places of misery, both for the animals and for the humans, beloved creatures of a God who declared them good, who certainly hears their cries of anguish, and who specifically commands justice for immigrants and for the poor:

> You shall not withhold the wages of poor and needy laborers, whether other Israelites or aliens who reside in your land in one of your towns. (Deut 24:14)

> You know the heart of an alien, for you were aliens in the land of Egypt. (Ex 23:9)

> Those who oppress the poor insult their Maker,
>   but those who are kind to the needy honor him.
>   (Prov 14:31)

> Oppressing the poor in order to enrich oneself,
>   and giving to the rich, will lead only to loss. (Prov 22:16)

Jim Wallis of *Sojourners* is fond of retelling the story of the time he and his colleagues cut every verse from the Bible that talked about the oppressed and needy. It made a good hollow book when they were done. I haven't done a biblical excision with respect to food, but I suspect the results would be similarly enlightening.

RUTH AS A STORY OF FOOD JUSTICE

When I was fourteen, I read a Focus on the Family *Brio* magazine story about the Old Testament book of Ruth. The message of this little magazine story—echoed in books like *Power to Faith, Family, and Getting a Guy* and *Lady in Waiting*—centered on the supposed romance between Ruth and Boaz, the lesson being that single women and girls should find ways to serve God while they wait for "Mr. Right."[35] But the whole idea of romance wasn't around for a good two thousand years until after the book of Ruth was written, and Ruth's actual behavior—much more than keeping busy between husbands—is way off from any evangelical dating guidebook (she lies down by Boaz when he's asleep, for example). But both Ruth and Boaz far exceed and redefine the law's expectations with regard to justice, kindness and reconciliation. And food is at the center of it all.[36]

A childless widowhood is tragic in any context, but in the ancient world, it could mean anything from consignment to a life of prostitution or slavery to a sentence of death. Bereft of both sons and husband, Naomi, an older woman, faces almost certain starvation. Her daughters-in-law, also widowed, are still young enough to remarry, and she encourages them to do so. But Ruth, with a determined kindness that goes beyond any law, binds herself to Naomi with a commitment as strong as any marriage vow:

> Where you go, I will go;
>   where you lodge, I will lodge;
> your people shall be my people,
>   and your God my God. (Ruth 1:16)

Having previously fled Bethlehem because of famine, Ruth and
Naomi hear that "the LORD had visited His people in giving them
food" (Ruth 1:6 NASB) and choose to return. Even still, the two
women are extremely poor; they survive by gathering food from
the edges of the fields of people better off than they are, in accordance with the laws in Leviticus and Deuteronomy, which all
"work against the emergence of the poor as a class":[37]

> When you reap the harvest of your land, you shall not reap to
> the very edges of your field, or gather the gleanings of your
> harvest; you shall leave them for the poor and for the alien: I
> am the LORD your God. (Lev 23:22; see also 19:9; Deut 24:19)

When Ruth goes to glean, she "just so happens upon" a field belonging to a relative of Naomi: Boaz. Asking around about her, Boaz
learns of Ruth's devotion to her mother-in-law and responds with generosity going beyond any law's requirement: "Stay in my fields, drink
my water" he urges her, promising also a measure of protection—"I've
warned my young men not to touch you" (see Ruth 2:8-9).

It might seem like Boaz is flirting with Ruth, but his actions
toward her are probably better described as *hospitality*. The law
doesn't require him to tell his workers to leave out extra grain for
her, but he does. In fact, the law would have permitted Boaz to
exclude Ruth: she's a Moabite, as the text reminds us repeatedly,
and her ancestors refused to give hospitality in the form of bread
and water to the Israelites as they left Egypt. This insult led to a
prohibition against the Moabites:

> No . . . Moabite shall be admitted to the assembly of the
> LORD. Even to the tenth generation [Hebrew-Bible-speak for
> "*Seriously, not ever!*"], none of their descendants shall be ad-
> mitted to the assembly of the LORD. (Deut 23:3)

But Boaz doesn't say, "Oh, hey, I'm sorry for your bad situation,
Ruth, but your ancestors insulted mine, so I'm biblically required

to do the same to you." No. He breaks a law to fulfill the law with even greater kindness than that law required. Ruth and Boaz do what God does, what God *loves* to do—they share bread.

This trumps everything.

Subtly, Boaz's generosity in the form of grain foreshadows his greater generosity. Boaz marries Ruth and (if you'll forgive the pun—it's the Bible's, not mine) shares his seed in an even more fruitful way: Ruth has a baby, a son to redeem the ancestral land of Ruth's first husband, which secures Naomi's future. Ruth's kindness to Naomi is lavish: she was free to marry whomever she wished (a "younger man," Boaz suggested, hinting that maybe he was a bit too old); marrying Boaz was *for Naomi's benefit.*

When Ruth approaches Boaz to propose marriage, she also asks him to put his garment over her. This isn't nearly as risqué as you may suppose. It's more like, "Spread your wings over me"—an echo of the blessing Boaz gave Ruth earlier:

> May you have a full reward from the LORD, the God of Israel, under whose wings you have come for refuge! (Ruth 2:12)

Boaz's wings, God's wings—this comparison suggests that Boaz does God's work. He agrees to be the one to protect Ruth. And Ruth, too, seems to understand that the God of Israel's work is carried out also by the hands of God's people—not least by *her.*

As God has given bread directly, so again God gives something else directly: conception, resulting in a baby, Obed, "a restorer of life and a nourisher of . . . old age" to his grandmother (Ruth 4:15)—who becomes the grandfather of David, from whose family line came Jesus, the Bread of Life for all the world.

FEEDING THE HUNGRY

In light of Ruth, we might understand our obligation to feed the hungry as carrying out God's own work. Offering food to the foreigner— yes, even to the illegal immigrant!—is an act of righteousness.[38]

But what can we do? The system that I've just barely described is immense and powerful; perhaps you, like me, feel overwhelmed at the very thought of large-scale greed and abuse.

How *can* we "eat with joy" when so much suffering and injustice exists, seemingly at every level of modern food production?

The first thing to do is open our ears, eyes and hearts to the stories of people who are poor. If you are not poor, have never been poor or have not known any poor people, it's difficult to understand what it's really like to run out of paycheck before you run out of month but not of food.

As the Proverb says:

The righteous know the rights of the poor;
     the wicked have no such understanding. (Prov 29:7)

Stopping at mere intellectual knowledge of poverty doesn't do anyone much good. The Hebrew word for "know" goes beyond the English translation to encompass the idea of intimate understanding, implying involvement. It's appropriate to include in our mealtime graces a prayer for the people whose work brought food to our plates. If we hold them in our minds and bring them before God, we will not remain numb to their suffering and eat the fruits of their labor in ignorance.

It's also good idea to find, when possible, foods that have come from places of joy. This can be difficult, but often it's as easy as finding a farmer's market or joining a CSA (community-supported agriculture) program, where you can meet the person who picked your vegetables or slaughtered your chicken. As with the open-air slaughterhouse (and as our grandmothers warned us not to buy ground beef from butchers who grind "behind closed doors"), visibility means accountability. Knowing who is bringing you food will also motivate you to see that it comes to you in a way that honors God and God's beloved creatures.

The Internet is a powerful tool in learning about your food and making ethical choices: a quick search for "food justice" or "fair food" will lead you to many helpful resources. Many blogs exist to point consumers toward food that is healthfully and fairly produced. The Christian organization Bread for the World lobbies on behalf of people who are hungry both in the US and abroad; their publications are enormously informative. By keeping informed on the issues surrounding the politics of food—food lobbying, federal nutrition standards and the Farm Bill—you can make wise choices in your own purchasing as well as influence the democratic process by petitioning for greater corporate responsibility and legislation that helps protect our neighbors who are most vulnerable.[39]

The activist and new monastic Shane Claiborne tells a story about when he first moved into the Kensington neighborhood of Philadelphia. "It's easier to get a gun in this neighborhood than it is to get a salad," a child told him. But today, that's no longer true. The Simple Way community has planted gardens in Jesus' name amid the empty lots and concrete jungle that is Philadelphia, bringing fresh food to the "food desert" and testifying to the God who loves gardens as well as cities: "The [biblical] story ends in Revelation with the image of the garden taking over the City of God, with the river of life flowing through the city center and the tree of life piercing the urban concrete."[40]

Explore your own eating habits in light of your neighbors, both local and global, so that you may work in ways appropriate to you and your situation toward eating that is "joyful though you have considered all the facts."[41] In practical terms, I try to spend my money in ways that do not increase the wealth of the major fast-food chains. When my family eats out, we do our best to eat in independently owned establishments. I'm willing—when I can—to spend extra to support companies that, to the best of my understanding, are respectable in their business practices. And I cook and bake "from scratch" as much as I can, partly because it's easier to figure out the natural history of what you're eating when you make it yourself, as opposed to when you buy and eat food that is already prepared.

But there are many people who, for reasons involving time, money and education, can't make such choices. How can those of us who have choices create possibilities for all to be better fed? On a broader level, it's reasonable to support your representatives in ending government subsidies on "commodity crops"—the corn and soybeans that are processed into the ingredients for sodas and chips—or at least to level the playing field and offer similar support to farmers producing foods eaten largely in their field-to-plate state, like vegetables and fruits. In 2009, for example, just 5 percent of federal farm subsidies supported the production of fresh produce. The vast majority of subsidies helped produce the very food that's making so many of us sick and overweight and hurting workers in the meantime.

On a smaller scale, you could support a local food pantry in offering healthier, fresher foods that are culturally appropriate to the people you serve.[42] My church's food pantry serves mainly people who have come to the US from Latin America. Generally speaking, they have much less use for boxed macaroni and cheese than for plain canned or dry beans and *masa harina*, a corn flour used for making tortillas. Additionally, grassroots efforts like offering free cooking classes for children and adults in otherwise-unused church kitchens can help make from-scratch cooking a possibility for more people. Various studies have demonstrated the effectiveness of basic cooking instruction in improving the quality of people's diets while keeping grocery costs down.

In the faces of immigrant workers, people who are poorly fed in our own communities, families that can't afford much beyond the cheapest offerings of the dollar store and Walmart, and hungry children whose village has Coke but not clean water, we must see Jesus and serve him as Ruth and Boaz would have—with greater generosity, creativity and love than "law" requires.[43]

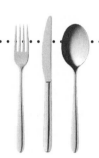

PRAYERS BEFORE EATING

God of the just weight
and the fair measure,
let me remember the hands
that harvested my food, my drink,
not only in my prayers
but in the marketplace.
Let me not seek a bargain
That leaves another hungry.[44]

For food in a world where many walk in hunger;
For faith in a world where many walk in fear;
For friends in a world where many walk alone;
We give you thanks, O Lord. Amen.[45]

O God,
Bless this food we are about to receive.
Give bread to those who are hungry
And make we who have bread
To hunger for justice.
Nicaraguan Prayer

May God bless those who eat, and may he bless all those who worked to bring this food to the table. To Christ, who feeds us, be all glory, forever. Amen.
Armenian Prayer[46]

RECIPES

No-Frills Lentil Soup

Lentils are widely touted as the convenience food of the legume family since they don't require presoaking or precooking. However, I think presoaking and precooking renders them both tastier and more digestible. I grew up on this soup. It's about as simple and inexpensive as recipes get and gets rave reviews whenever I make it.

Start by rinsing and soaking **1 pound green (most of us think of them as brown) lentils** in fresh water to cover. Soak for at least 1 hour, then drain and rinse again. Cover with fresh water, bring to a boil, then simmer for 1 hour.

Meanwhile, heat a soup pot over medium heat and cover the bottom with **about ¼ cup olive oil**. (You really must use olive oil—in a soup this simple, each ingredient has a lot of work to do.) Add **1 or 2 large yellow onions, finely chopped**, and **1 tablespoon minced garlic**. Cook these for 10 minutes, stirring constantly, then add the **cooked, drained lentils** and **1 tablespoon ground cumin**. Stir for 1 minute more, then add a quart or so of cold water. Bring to a boil; simmer for 45 minutes, adding about **2 teaspoons salt** and some **fresh black pepper**. Stir in **fresh juice squeezed from 1 lemon** and taste again to adjust for saltiness and acidity. Remove from heat, drizzle in a bit more olive oil and serve alongside bowls of plain steamed rice or slices of fresh bread.

Dilly Cucumber Salad

This recipe reminds me of our family's year spent living in Germany. There, this would be called *guerkensalaet*. It's delicious—reminiscent of pickles but much fresher. Quick and easy to prepare, it's really best in spring and summer with seasonal cucumbers—imported ones won't give you the best flavor.

Thinly slice **3 cucumbers**, toss with **2 tablespoons fresh chopped dill (or 2 teaspoons dried), 1 clove garlic, minced, 3 tablespoons red wine vinegar, 1 tablespoon olive oil** and **1/2 teaspoon sugar**.

. . . .

POINTS FOR ACTION

- Learn about hunger relief programs in your own community and get involved in ways that help elevate the dignity, health and joy of those who depend on such programs.

- Save money on your food redemptively. If you eat out a lot, eat more meals at home; if you eat a lot of expensive meals at home, choose to simplify more of your meals in solidarity with those for whom simplicity is a requirement.

- Encourage your church to hold a "hunger banquet" or to participate in World Vision's 30-Hour Famine.

- Avoid food snobbery. An alternative to fussiness might be gratitude for what you have and generosity toward those who don't have the resources you do.

- Get to know some of the people who produce your food. If you can, become one of them! Even growing some herbs in a flowerpot is a good start toward connecting more mindfully with the food you eat.

3

Communal Eating

HOW MEALS BRING US TOGETHER

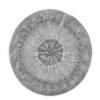

A meal eaten in solitude isn't always a bad thing.

In my busy house, where meals are raucous affairs with many people talking at once and children bargaining over what they do and do not want to eat, I sometimes relish the chance to eat quietly by myself, perhaps in the company of a good book or my laptop, browsing blogs as I eat.

But this strange luxury is made possible only by modern conveniences. In ages past, there would have been no question of lighting the fire just to prepare one small meal or to heat up some leftovers for one person's snack. Pilot-lit stoves, refrigerators and microwaves (not to mention single-serve frozen dishes and other prepared foods) have made eating alone easy where once it wasn't.

I've always hated seeing people eat alone in a restaurant. The solo diners I served as a waitress sometimes wanted to be left alone, but more often they wanted to talk to me. Eating out, rather than at home, was maybe "less alone" for them, talking to the waitress better than talking to no one. People are made for community, and part of that means *eating* in community.

Anthropologists and biologists have persuasively argued that food and its preparation are the foundations of families and even of cultures—to get enough calories, hunter-gatherers would have had to have some kind of division of labor, with hunters killing meat and others cooking it.[1] The humorous documentary *How Beer Saved the World* shows how agriculture formed the basis of human culture, with the preparation, sharing and exchange of grain (in the form of beer) laying the foundations for art, law and economics, to say nothing of the culinary arts and the traditions of the table.

Every culture values food as a "powerful social component,"[2] in ways ranging from the highly ceremonial to the everyday. In some places it's considered inappropriate for a couple engaged to be married to eat with one another before the wedding. The traditional feeding that is part of the wedding ceremony is, in those contexts, a powerful indication of the couple's unity, commitment and promise to mutual care. Sharing food non-ceremonially is an important indication of welcome and friendship in virtually every culture,[3] whether it's beverages, nuts or, as I experienced in France, some cheese or an apéritif. "Let's meet for coffee," we say to a new acquaintance we hope to get to know better.

Our English word *companion* comes from the Latin for "with" (*com*) and "bread" (*panis*)—a companion is one with whom you eat your bread. Food being as importantly generative of relationships as it is to bodily growth, eating together is a universally important human activity. Think about the way food plays a role even at seemingly non-food-related events like a book club meeting—food provides a gathering point, a center around which to build relationships and trust. Jesus seemed to attribute particular significance to shared meals as well—his table fellowship forms an important part of the Gospels and, extended by his followers, a vital part of the church's common life.[4]

Especially in the first three Gospels, Jesus is seen eating frequently with all kinds of questionable characters, which earned him the criticism of the Pharisees: "Why does he eat with tax collectors and sinners?" (Mk 2:16). These meals with sinners, "an expression of [their] new relationship with Jesus,"[5] recur throughout the Gospels. Further, Jesus teaches his followers to do as he did: to welcome as guests at a banquet "the poor, the crippled, the lame, and the blind" (Lk 14:13), precisely those who would be able give back *nothing* to the host in terms of worldly benefits or prestige.

This invitation to the banquet isn't a handout or a ticket for the soup kitchen line. It's an invitation to share a common table, a vision that is most certainly an extension of Mosaic law. In his sermon on Deuteronomy 15, John Calvin writes:

> As God bestoweth his benefites upon us, let us beware that wee acknowledge it towardes him, by doing good to our neighbors whome he offereth unto us, so as wee neither exempt ourselves from their want, nor seclude them from our abundance, but gently make them partakers with us, as folke that are linked together in an inseparable bond.[6]

Eating together was an important aspect of the early church's common life—a powerful symbol of unity both with Christ and with one another. Eating *with* the poorest, the weakest and the most vulnerable is an essential aspect of those early Communion meals, a point that's emphasized in the famous 1 Corinthians 11 passage and hinted at in James's epistle.

For Jesus, eating with sinners and other unsavory folk was not merely symbolic. It was a way of tangibly practicing the kind of peace, equality and unity that he proclaimed. And he urged his followers that there would be true blessing and reward from doing the same, encouraging open fellowship where it was once unthinkable—Gentiles could eat with Jews!

In Acts 10, Peter is hungry and wants something to eat, but

the people he is with are "unclean" because of their work as tanners. Going up on the roof to pray, the Spirit of Jesus gives him a vision, telling him that God has made all food clean. Though he's kept kosher all his life, prompted by Christ's Spirit, Peter goes to the house of a Gentile, Cornelius, to have table fellowship with him and to tell him the good news of racial and ethnic equality in Jesus:

> Then Peter began to speak to them: "I truly understand that God shows no partiality, but in every nation anyone who fears him and does what is right is acceptable to him." (Acts 10:34-35)

It is perhaps a bit difficult for us to grasp how radical this was: Peter was giving up his lifelong foodways—tantamount to his very identity—for the sake of Christ, unifying himself with those whom he'd always regarded as "unclean." Powerful stuff indeed! It's about as shocking as it would be to see a vegan chef sitting down to eat chili dogs with Paula Deen, or, as Philip Yancey says, as radical as an alcohol-stocked bar descending into a gathering of Southern Baptists, with a voice from heaven saying, "Drink!"[7]

Early Christian writers claimed that sharing life, including meals, with persons of different backgrounds was a "proof" of true Christian faith. They were convinced that practicing the broadly open hospitality that Jesus taught meant that they would welcome Christ himself as their guest—as, of course, Christ himself teaches in Matthew 25—and that their actions would "portray a clear message—that of equality, transformed relations, and a common life."[8]

Yet, according to theologian Christine Pohl, the Christian habit of sharing meals regularly and with "the least of these" all but disappeared as a significant moral practice relatively early on in the life of the church.[9] Today, if churches feed those who are poor, it's usually done in the context of ministries like soup kitchens and food pantries. It is the rare group that—like the L'Arche communities founded by Jean Vanier—regularly practices sharing meals across the boundaries of social class, background and, in L'Arche homes, intellectual capability. It's precisely this kind of sharing that comes closest to Jesus' ideal.

When I was in junior high, a half dozen or so adults with intellectual disabilities who shared a house began attending our church regularly, and they invited my family over for dinner: baked ziti, garlic bread and salad. As the only daughter of a pastor, I'd been to a lot of boring, "let's impress the Reverend with our piety" kinds of dinners. *This* meal was anything but boring. Seeing adults who needed help cutting and eating their food and even, in some cases, who needed bibs was fascinating, if slightly uncomfortable for a twelve-year-old. But mostly I remember a lot of laughter and so much happiness that we had come over. I even thought: *It's almost as if they're having a permanent sleep over; they're all friends, and they get to live together.* I can't remember another meal where the hosts were so overjoyed at our mere presence. After lunch, there was singing and pulling out photo albums, and Alan, the man with cerebral palsy in addition to a form of intellectual limitation, told us how much he loved Paul McCartney, so much that he felt like he *was* Paul McCartney. "See?" he said, pointing to a picture of the beloved Beatle. Then, conspiratorially, "That's *me*." No one wanted us to leave. There were lots of hugs, smiles and calls of "Please, please come again!"

• •

"Each day brings with it not only the necessity of eating but the renewal of our love of and in God."

—Kathleen Norris, *The Quotidian Mysteries*

• •

Pohl writes, "Meal time, when people sit down together, is the clearest time of being *with* others, rather than doing *for* others."[10]

After all, it wasn't until Jesus broke bread that Cleopas and the unnamed disciple recognized his resurrection body. There's a different dynamic going on when I serve my kids some pasta and veggies before I leave them with their grandparents and go out, as opposed to when I spend hours making roast chicken, a salad, corn on the cob, fresh rolls and lemonade, and we all sit down to take in the savory and buttery and yeasty fragrances and all the crunchy, sour, soft, salty, cooling flavors and textures *together*. We sit at the same time, at the same table, acknowledging our common creatureliness as we stop and do the necessary, joyful business of eating. The same food goes into each of our bodies, building up our cells, becoming, quite literally, a part of each of us. We make memories and get a little closer to one another as we laugh and talk. A memorable meal might even come up weeks later: *Remember when we ate that thing with the noodles?* Sometimes table chatter is nonstop; sometimes the only sounds are of contented chewing. But regardless, we're mysteriously bound to each other in the breaking of bread.

And Christ is with us.

But shared meals of *any* kind are on the decline. It's normal for people to eat alone and on the run. A few years ago, a BBC article reported that half of all meals eaten in the UK are eaten *alone*.[11] Not only are there more and more single-person households, but ready-to-eat meals—like TV dinners, except not necessarily frozen—are affordable and *everywhere*. I don't know how many meals are eaten alone in the US, but there's no shortage of research reporting a steady decline in the number of meals that children eat with their parents. A few years ago, barely a third of teenagers ate with their parents six or seven times each week, and another third ate with their parents fewer than three times each week.[12]

If eating together is so much a part of being human, and if extending our tables to those who are different from us is such an essential part of living Jesus' good news, what can it mean for our overall health—spiritual, physical and emotional—that even shared *family* meals are on the decline?

MOSTLY ALONE

Spoiler Alert *The following discussion gives away significant plot information about the German film* Mostly Martha. *If you haven't seen the film, you may want to skip ahead until you've had a chance to watch it!*

In the German film *Mostly Martha*, the brilliant chef Martha Klein is professionally meticulous but personally a mess. She's enraged when customers critique her food, short-tempered and exacting with her kitchen staff, and aloof. Multiple times throughout her shift, she retreats to the walk-in refrigerator to cool off both body and temper. At the behest of the restaurant owner, she attends weekly therapy sessions, during which she refuses to discuss what she's thinking and feeling, instead subjecting her therapist to detailed descriptions of her culinary creations. Sometimes she even cooks for her therapist, despite his protests and consternation: "If you would sit and eat with me, Martha, I'd be able to think that we're making some progress."

But she won't.

We don't see Martha eat *anything* for the first half of the film. She's present at the table but is reading—not eating or conversing—while the other restaurant staff are enjoying their meal. When she cooks herself a beautiful dinner at home, she doesn't eat it. Sitting down to eat, she notices music coming from the apartment below and goes downstairs to greet her new neighbor and offer him something to eat. "Are you inviting me to dinner?" he asks with a wry smile. "No!" she exclaims, adding, "but I could bring you something to eat if you're hungry." He politely declines, adding that he's interested in getting together with *her* another time. She can offer food but not a relationship— not even companionship.

Martha's isolation is highlighted when she becomes guardian of her eight-year-old niece following an accident in which Martha's sister is killed. Visiting her niece in the hospital after the car crash, a doctor reports to Martha that Lina hasn't been eating. Martha glances at Lina's unappetizing hospital meal tray and promises to make her the best meal she's ever had after she gets out of the hospital. Lina senses what Martha is unable to say and asks: "Is mom dead?" Martha replies, "Yes," and Lina turns to the wall. Not another word passes between them.

Lina comes to live with Martha, skulking around in grief and despair, saying nothing, eating nothing. When babysitting arrangements fall through one evening, Lina ends up hanging out in the kitchen of Martha's restaurant. By this time, Martha is frantic over Lina's hunger strike, saying so under her breath. The new kitchen assistant, Mario, whose voluble and enthusiastic ways Martha disdains, overhears and, with a bit of friendliness, gets Lina to eat. Thus begins her (and Martha's) return to health.

Lina asks Martha if they can have Mario over for dinner. Martha reluctantly agrees. "I'll cook," she says. "No," Lina replies, "I want *him* to cook. . . . I prefer Italian food." The evening comes, and, as promised, Lina and Mario do all the food preparation, locking Martha out of the kitchen. Mario makes a huge mess—it's so bad that Martha hyperventilates when she peeks in—preparing a delicious feast that the three of them share from common dishes while sitting on a picnic blanket. (This is the first time we see Martha eat *anything.*) After Lina falls asleep, we sense a growing attraction between Martha and Mario. When he leaves, Martha cleans up the kitchen disaster and does something totally out of character—she returns to the refrigerator, eats a spoonful of dessert straight from the dish and *smiles.*

From there Martha learns to eat with—and to love—other people. In the penultimate scene, she's back at therapy, eating a piece of cake that her therapist made for *her.* Unlike before, they are sitting on the therapy couch *together*, on the same level. She has become well.

Eating with others is more than just a symbol of friendship, of belonging, of mutual trust—it is a living metaphor for our connection with other human beings as well as our dependence on the God who feeds us. In her memoir *The Tapestry*, Edith Schaeffer wrote that in the early years of their marriage, when Francis was a seminary student and she worked from home as a seamstress, she packed identical lunches for each of them every day, even though she wasn't going to leave their apartment. She explains that she wanted to taste the same flavors that her husband would be tasting and wanted to feel the "same degree of hunger by dinnertime." Eating the same lunch, even separately, was for them a way of "being together even when apart."[13] Not only is there a sense of conviviality—of joyful fellowship—when eating with others, there is also the reality of meeting physical needs together, of seeing that the other has enough, of nourishing each other with bread and fruit and companionship. You can be a James Beard award-winning chef and miss this about food—that it's all about creating and sustaining *relationships*.

FOOD AND FAMILIES AND BEYOND

My father is one of the small fraction of Americans who have Celiac disease, a lifelong intolerance to wheat, barley and other grains. That means things like bread, pizza, cake, cookies and pasta are toxic to him, as well as less obvious things like beer, soy sauce and bouillon. It's an easily managed condition, but what my dad misses even more than New York pizza is being able to eat whatever everyone else is eating. There's almost nothing you can eat at Italian restaurants or at Super Bowl parties or at potlucks, and you have the uncomfortable obligation of explaining—without getting into messy gastrointestinal details—why you can't eat this or that when you're eating with friends. My dad still gets misty-eyed when he remembers how the older ladies in his congregation—mostly now either deceased or too old to cook—tweaked their time-worn recipes to make them gluten-free, making little toothpicked signs reading "For Pastor" at church potlucks. On the other hand, he recalls with pain how he always felt unwelcome in his father and stepmother's house, where they never accommodated his diet. He had to fill up on lettuce or chips or something while everyone ate the "real" meal.

When we eat together, I try really hard to make a meal that includes everyone—if we're having pasta, I cook regular pasta *and* the gluten-free variety, even taking care to match the shapes (spaghetti with spaghetti, penne with penne and so forth) so that my dad's meal, if it must be different, will look much like everyone else's. Silly? Maybe a little. But maybe I take Nora Ephron seriously when she says: "A family is a group of people who eat the same thing for dinner."[14]

A growing body of evidence suggests that the solitary eating trend may in fact be highly detrimental in all kinds of measurable (and immeasurable) ways. When people eat alone, they tend to overeat or eat too little, to eat food that is of poorer quality and to enjoy it less. Books like *The Surprising Power of Family Meals* by Miriam Weinstein and *The Family Dinner* by Laurie David emphasize research findings from numerous sources showing that the more meals children eat with their families, the better off they are. Kids eating with their families regularly not only eat a much more balanced and healthy diet, they also do better in school, have more satisfying peer relationships, are less inclined to develop eating disorders, and are less likely to use drugs, tobacco and alcohol.

Given the life-giving nature of table fellowship in every culture, is it any wonder that throughout the history of Christianity, the shared meal has been "central to every community . . . central to sustaining the life of the community and expressing welcome to strangers"?[15] If we are to follow Jesus' example and exhortation to feed those in need, it might be best to begin at home, using meals as a base from which to connect with those we live with and then to reach out to others, to give them a place to belong. But in the Gospels and the book of Acts, the family of God that's formed by following Jesus involves loving brothers and sisters and mothers and fathers and children that aren't our relatives *as if they were our own*, which certainly should include sharing meals.

In her biography of the Obamas, Jodi Kantor points out that even President Obama refused to miss dinner with his family more than two nights a week; "barring special circumstances, that was the most he was willing to tolerate being away from his family." Trips, galas, fundraising and "working dinners" were trumped by sitting down to a meal with Michelle, Sasha and Malia.[16] If the leader of the free world is willing to turn down politically and socially advantageous engagements in favor of more time at the table with his wife and children, I suspect that many of us could manage similar readjustments. (Granted, most of us don't have a personal chef cooking for us each night, but most of us aren't the commander in chief of the world's largest economic and military power either.) It's also true that children today have many of their own extracurricular commitments, but it is possible to schedule the dinner hour several nights a week as an event of equal or greater importance than other activities, to be worked around rather than "squeezed in."

There are many things that happen around the table that can't happen anywhere else. Perhaps more than anything, it's the place where children absorb the message: *These are my people, and I belong here.* It's sort of the family Eucharistic table, the daily sacrament of being united to one another and to God in the breaking of bread.

RECOGNIZING THE BODY

I always thought that Paul's famous Communion passage in 1 Corinthians 11—"For all who eat and drink without discerning the body, eat and drink judgment against themselves" (v. 29)—had something to do with understanding that the bread and wine were not "just" bread and wine but actually represented Christ's body. So, judgment would be on you if you just grabbed for the bread and wine, eating and drinking as if it was any ordinary snack and drink, almost as if you were a bumbling character in a fairy tale eating the magic apple intended for someone else.

But in fact this passage has more to do with eating *together*. "Come on, church," Paul is saying, "some of you are pigging out and getting drunk while others are lucky just to get a crust of bread." The profanity was in the lack of sharing and in the shaming of the poor folks who had little or nothing to bring. "This *isn't* the Lord's Supper," Paul says, "because this isn't what Jesus is about." Jesus says that his friends must share with other people; that satisfying our neighbor's hunger and thirst is at least as important—maybe more important—than satisfying our own. It's not an ethic that's easily compatible with the "meal for one" society. Eating with Jesus requires sharing. It requires making room—real and symbolic—for hungry people.

It's possible in our contemporary context to reclaim the ancient and universal practice of sharing meals so as to proclaim the peace and hope and reconciliation promised in Christ's death, burial and resurrection. Eating is something we all have to make time for anyway—doing so *with others* takes a bit more imagination and creativity than perhaps it once did, but it's still within reach for most of us. As an expression of Christian welcome and hospitality, I can think of nothing quite like a shared meal. It's why we bring food to people who are hurting, who have lost someone or who have undergone surgery. It's why we invite stray children in for dinner. I even know someone who invited their lonely UPS driver to share a meal.

In a culture that runs on food as fuel, always trying to make it faster, cheaper, more profitable and less communal—I recently read an op-ed piece on schoolchildren who were allotted just ten minutes to eat lunch at school—it can be profoundly countercultural to practice regularly the kind of meals that have existed from the dawn of humanity—meals that take some time, thought and care to prepare, meals drawn from sources that are sustainable and nourishing, and meals that are eaten in joyful, caring conviviality. We can hardly hope to realize Christ's ideal of extending our tables to "the least of these" irrespective of race, class and background if we are not regularly nourishing ourselves and those nearest to us—often, our families—with a satisfying rhythm of shared eating.

But while I believe that it's crucial to establish a regular routine of family meals, I'd rather not stop there and call it enough. I believe Jesus calls us to more than that, to look around and find people who need someone to eat with—a lonely elderly person, perhaps, or someone suffering with an eating disorder who needs love and feeding and listening, and more love and feeding.

For several months before he died, I brought my friend Jack a steak dinner every Saturday night. He was ninety-one, and while people will say that old people don't have sensitive taste buds anymore, Jack hated the food and coffee at the nursing home. All his life, he took great pleasure in hearty meals of steak, black coffee and some kind of rich chocolate dessert. So that's what I brought him. He needed company, and he needed to know that even though he was near death, he was still alive. I fussed over those meals, perfected cream sauces and chocolate mousse, and lugged them into the nursing home on china dishes. And then we would sit together in the low-slung, fluorescent-lit, antiseptic-and-urine-scented nursing home and savor the goodness of food and of company. I could almost smell Jesus' perfumed feet readied for burial right there with us as we ate.

In our community of theological students in St. Andrews, Scotland, there were babies being born all the time. (After all, many of us were American, and the chance to have a "free" baby on the National Health Service was too good to pass up.) Each family with a new baby received a month of meals every other night as soon as the baby was born, courtesy of the other families in the community, an arrangement made beforehand via email. (Websites like MealTrain.com make this kind of ministry even easier.) I'll never forget the evening when my husband was away coaching basketball and both of our children— the two-year-old and the new baby—were bawling, when my friend Cheng Ping showed up with a huge dish of stir-fried rice and vegetables. The compassion and care in her eyes were every bit as nourishing as the delicious food.

When my husband and I lived in a tiny town in rural California, pastoring an even tinier church, we helped establish a tradition of twice-monthly potlucks. In such an isolated place, most people desperately needed excuses to get together. It was too easy for everyone to stay home idling in front of the television, forgetting how to live in community. So we had potlucks. Ethel, who was ninety-two, brought the same pea salad every time. Judy made potato casseroles that I think were largely crafted by mixing things from cans, bottles and boxes. And there was always some kind of glowing neon molded Jell-O salad that Tim and I pretended to taste. The meals became such a hit that even those people who wouldn't come to church services began showing up after the final hymn with casserole dishes in hand. The needs those meals met were legion. Some of the people who came didn't often get enough to eat; some didn't get enough human contact; some—grandmas whose loved ones all lived far away—didn't get enough opportunities to serve and fuss over and clean up after other people. There were awkward moments (like one week where everyone brought dessert) and weird dishes and too much Cool Whip, but those meals were served and eaten and cleaned up with so much love, so much gratitude and so much joy that I know for sure that Jesus couldn't help but drop in from time to time.

I know that most of us have—or, at the least, *think* we have— obstacles that keep us from eating with others. People live alone, people live with roommates with odd schedules, people have no time for cooking, people have messy houses and greasy, crumby stovetops. It can feel vulnerable and awkward to invite other people to your house to eat with you. Going out to a restaurant and splitting the bill is easier than the old-fashioned "we'd like to have you over for dinner."

But eating with others and inviting people over and cooking for them in your house are things worth doing, and here's why: be- cause we need to take turns being guest and host, like Jesus did. We need to go to awkward meals at other awkward people's messy houses and have people over to our awkward, messy houses be- cause that's where grace comes to us—in the awkwardness and in the mess.

It's not that I'm keen to have guests see my home in its natural, Lego-strewn state. I'd love for everything and everyone to be clean, tidy and perfect before guests come. I don't want them to see a dirty dish or a dirty dishcloth and think that maybe the food's not going to be very sanitary. I don't want them to know that I'm not very strict about insisting that my children put away one set of toys before getting out another, or that I let them eat apples or crackers while they play or read. I'd like to give off the impression that I've got things together—that it was simply a breeze for me to whip up that glorious meal while my children played neatly and quietly among my gleaming rooms.

The truth is, though, that I don't like it at all when I feel like people are trying to impress me with their perfect life or house or kids; it makes me afraid that if they really get to know me, my life, my house and my kids, they won't like me. When my husband and I realized that we wanted to marry each other, we took turns telling each other our deepest, darkest secrets—the things we most wanted to keep hidden—because if there's anything we all *need,* it's to be known and accepted as we are so that, as the apostle Paul says, grace may abound. That can't really happen if you keep yourself at a distance from your guests by staging a perfect show loosely based on your real life. I'm not saying don't clean the house or cook something nice. I'm saying that if you offer a warm and authentic welcome in Jesus' name, you're likely to make a *friend*—and *be* one too.

Once my friend Ruth, who lived alone, invited us over for lentil stew that had been simmering all day, but when it came time to eat, we realized that the lentils were still hard: they had had a very, very long life on the shelf of her dry California pantry, and it turned out that they were pretty much dead. Ruth was embarrassed at first, but we quickly saw the funny side of things, improvised some waffles and fruit salad and went on with the feast. If your dinner plans turn disastrous—the oven stayed cold or the stew scorched through—shrug your shoulders and boil some water for spaghetti with sauce from a jar, or call in an order for take-out. Give yourself—and your guests— grace in the midst of the mild adversity of a failed beef roast, and they'll know that it's fellowship with them more than the quality of the food or your performance as a host that's important to you.

The grace we can extend to one another in Christian hospitality comes best when we stop trying to impress and compete with each other and instead accept that we are all the beneficiaries—and potential conduits of—wildly amazing grace. As the priest and amateur cook Robert Farrar Capon wrote, "Grace cannot prevail . . . until our lifelong certainty that someone is keeping score has run out of steam and collapsed."[17]

So don't wait until the bathroom remodel is finished, or until you have a chance to shampoo the carpet, or until you have time to plan and execute an impressive six-course menu. I live in a house that was built almost two hundred years ago, and almost nothing has been remodeled. There are bumps in the floor and on the walls, and the carpets are hideous. But not long ago I had a family over for dinner after church and served something utterly ordinary, like rice and beans, and Anna, the mom, settled into a worn, comfy chair and gave me the best compliment ever: "It feels peaceful here." (Which, to be fair, may have been due in part to the fact that my kids were sick with fevers upstairs, tucked into my bed watching PBS Kids on my laptop. In health, they're expert disturbers of peace. But you get the idea.)

Martha Stewart and the Food Network—moneymaking machines that they are—are always trying to persuade you that you have to put on a show for your guests and that you need whatever it is they're selling to do that. But what you could do is simply start with what you already know how to cook on an ordinary weeknight and invite some people over to share this ordinary meal with you. The point is not to impress—the goal is to *love your neighbor* in breaking bread together. And practicing hospitality is just that—*practicing!* The more you make and serve and share meals with your family and others, it becomes easier, more natural. We've had some guests over so many times that I assign them chopping and cleaning-up chores without a second thought. "You've been here three times now, so you're not a guest anymore," I'll say. "Now you're family, so grab a dishtowel."

When you put more extenders in your table than is exactly comfortable, you may just be surprised that Jesus shows up as a guest too.

· ·

PRAYERS BEFORE EATING

For all your gifts of nature and of grace,
For health and strength,
For homes and family
For true friends and wise teachers,
For all the blessings of this life and for our hope of a better life to
  come.
Amen.
Adapted from Good Graces, *based on a Church of Scotland prayer*

Come, Lord Jesus, be our guest,
May this food by you be blest,
May our souls by you be fed,
Always on the living Bread.
Amen.

Jesus said: "My food is to do the will of him who sent me" (Jn 4:34).

We thank you, God of creation,
For the food that nourishes bodies.
Give us also that food which compels us to do your will
And to share the fruits of creation among all;
Through Jesus Christ our Lord.
Amen.

Let us give thanks for the plenteous gifts of the Lord, our God,
Who feeds us day by day in abundance in his lovingkindness, so
  that

He may make us his servants as we wait and hope for the kingdom
of Heaven.

Amen.

Armenian Prayer

. . . .

RECIPES

Strawberry Rhubarb Pie

My mom was convinced that she didn't like rhubarb until I made
one of these pies for her, using fresh strawberries and rhubarb
from the farm stand we're lucky to have nearby. This changed
her mind forever about rhubarb; now she wants to grow some in
her garden.

It really helps to chill all the ingredients in the refrigerator for
1 hour before beginning the piecrust. And, yes—piecrusts are a
bit tricky, but the pre-made ones are loaded with scary ingredients, whereas this one's rich, but still *real*.

For the crust:
Combine in a small bowl and place in the refrigerator:
1 slightly beaten egg
5 tablespoons ice cold water
1 tablespoon vinegar (white or cider)

Meanwhile, in the bowl of a food processor, pulse together:
3 cups pastry flour (may use up to 1/3 whole wheat pastry
flour)
1 cup of very cold butter
1 teaspoon salt

Pour in the wet ingredients and pulse until a dough ball forms.
Cut into thirds and chill for half an hour; remove one ball at a
time and roll out gently on a floured surface. Each ball will yield
a single 9" piecrust; wrapped well, they can be frozen to use another time.

For the filling:
3 cups rhubarb, cut into small pieces
1 cup stemmed and sliced strawberries
1 cup raw (turbinado) sugar
2 tablespoons cornstarch
Squeeze of lemon juice
Dash of nutmeg (optional)
1/4 teaspoon salt

Combine well in a large bowl. Pour filling into prepared pie crust. Top with a second pie crust, and slit to allow steam to escape. Bake at 400° F for 20 minutes; lower heat to 350° and bake an additional 30-40 minutes. Cool in a pan on rack. The juices will thicken as the pie cools. Delicious served with vanilla ice cream or lightly sweetened whipped heavy cream.

Spring/Summer Rolls and Peanut Sauce

Oh, yumminess! When I first made these rolls for my dad, using fresh stuff from the farm stand, he couldn't stop eating them and exclaiming, "I can't believe how good these are! I can't believe how good these are!"

For the rolls:
8 sheets rice paper
8 soft lettuce leaves
4 ounces thin rice noodles, soaked until tender (but not mushy)

A quantity of vegetables:
Grated or julienned carrots, cucumber, avocado, radishes—be creative!

1/2 cup each fresh mint, cilantro and basil leaves torn into pieces
(If you lack one of these, feel free to omit.)

Soak 1 sheet of rice paper in warm water for 10 seconds or so, then lay out on a kitchen cloth. Place a lettuce leaf in the middle, and fill it with a finger-size portion of noodles, a bit of each vege-table and some of the fresh leaves. Roll up the rice-paper wrapper like a burrito, closing in both sides. Repeat with the remaining ingredients, making sure not to allow rolls to touch, or they will stick together. You can wrap them in a damp towel and plastic wrap and serve within an hour, with peanut sauce (my favorite) or a simple dipping sauce of equal parts soy sauce and rice vinegar with a couple tablespoons of sesame oil stirred in.

For the peanut sauce:
Chop finely and sauté together in 2-3 tablespoons of neutral oil (like corn or grapeseed) until tender and fragrant:
1 small onion
3 cloves garlic
1-inch piece ginger
1-2 stalks lemongrass (optional)

Sprinkle with 1 teaspoon turmeric and stir to coat, 1 minute. Then add:
1 can (organic, please!) coconut milk
2-3 tablespoons soy sauce
3 tablespoons brown or turbinado sugar (you can also use maple syrup; or substitute 1/4 cup hoisin sauce and reduce soy sauce to 1-2 tablespoons)
3 tablespoons fresh lime juice
1/2-1 cup non-hydrogenated peanut butter
Ground cayenne pepper to taste

Simmer, stirring constantly to keep from sticking and adding water to achieve the desired dipping consistency. Taste and adjust seasonings, and enjoy warm with spring/summer rolls and a dish of raw veggies. Cherry tomatoes taste fantastic dipped in this sauce. My kids love this dish. It's fun to eat and a great way to get lots of raw veggies into them.

● ●

POINTS FOR ACTION

- Be intentional and realistic about meal plans, and start with where you are. If you are currently eating only a few dinners a week as a family, try shooting for one or two more meals per week.

- Aim for one company meal per month and see how you do. Sometimes it's a good idea to have one "standard" guest meal. For a while, we had people over for crepes with fruit and whipped cream on Saturday mornings. Then it was Sunday afternoons, and we served spaghetti and meatballs. If you are making the same meal again and again, it becomes second nature.

- Invite old friends, of course, but also people that you wouldn't normally think to have over for a meal. Find someone who you know eats alone and invite them over or take a meal to them.

- Sometimes it's fun to *bring* dinner to someone's house and eat it with them. That way, only one of you has to cook, and only one of you has to clean.

4

Restorative Eating

HOW EATING TOGETHER HEALS

My friend Theresa grew up in a Catholic home on Long Island in the 1950s. She attended a local college so she could continue to live at home and avoid the expense of living on campus. Her mother cooked dinner every night, and when Theresa had to stay late for evening classes or club meetings, her mother would save a plate and have it warm and waiting on her return. Then they'd sit together while Theresa ate and her mother asked about her day. In that time and place, grabbing a bite to eat on the run between classes wasn't done. Her mother's cooking was neither especially fancy, nor what we might today consider especially healthy, but being able to rely on the family table gave Theresa a healthy confidence and pleasure in food that she retains even now.

When I was a college student living on campus, the all-you-can-eat, buffet-style, come-and-go character of the dining hall frightened me. Should I skip breakfast or lunch? What if I lost control and ate *way* too much? I wondered whether people were checking out my tray and judging me based on what was (or wasn't) on it. My stomach would be in knots before I even swiped my meal card. I'd frequently go to the bathroom before going into the cafeteria to wash my hands and check out my body in the mirror: *Was I ugly? Fat? Did I deserve a good meal, or did I deserve an abstemious tray of raw veggies and ice water?*

But when I moved in with my soon-to-be sister-in-law, Kym, I entered a different kind of eating culture. Sharing a house with a married couple and a baby—with many of our neighbors regularly dropping in to eat meals together—I no longer faced the anxieties of the cafeteria. And because Kym is a nurturing, caring person— and often expresses her care through *food*—she even packed my lunches sometimes. This was a gift to me. It speaks to the disorder of my thinking and behavior at the time that my reaction to the lunches she made was, *Wow! It's okay to eat lunch. It's okay to plan ahead for a good lunch.* Kym liked good food and liked feeding other people. Her confident, caring ways helped teach me to be unafraid of food. And it began with us enjoying food together, with her sending a bit of her love and concern to campus with me in a plaid L.L.Bean lunch bag.

Meals bring people together and help in all kinds of ways. Meals together are a wonderful "treatment" for boredom and loneliness, especially for the elderly and those who live alone; they also help stave off eating disorders. In contemporary Western cultures, that's no small recommendation.

EATING DISORDER NATION

For every person with an official diagnosis of anorexia nervosa, bulimia, binge-eating disorder, compulsive overeating or ED-NOS (eating disorder not otherwise specified), there are many more who struggle daily with feelings of addiction, revulsion, fear and anxiety surrounding their eating and their bodies—an anxiety I know from the inside. I'm not alone. Chances are good that you or someone you're close to also struggles with food. There are many reasons for this, not least among them our image-driven culture's obsession with extreme thinness. My friend Lisa, who teaches in a public high school, is diligent in educating her students about the artificiality of magazine images. In the 1960s, Lisa was very much a part of the counter-cultural movement, which is to say she may have burned a bras-siere or two and put in some serious time at protests, in com-munes and in a Volkswagen van. "I would've hoped that the liberation we were fighting for then would mean that these girls would be less anxious about their appearance today," Lisa told me. "But if anything, the obsession with physical perfection is worse today than it ever was before the sixties." A deeply com-mitted Christian, Lisa prays eagerly that her students would see their infinite value in God's eyes. And she demonstrates how Pho-toshop creates false images of women through various editing techniques. "We *know* it's fake," her students insist, "but we still want to look like that."

It doesn't help that images of extreme thinness are everywhere. Even the most seemingly mundane objects show the trend: the girl on the Morton Salt container or on the bottle of White Rock water is thinner than she was twenty or thirty or fifty years ago. My children's Candy Land game (made in 2010) shows highly ide-alized, thin female characters and muscular male characters, whereas in the 1984 version I grew up playing the characters were, if anything, a little chubby. Similarly, toys like Strawberry Shortcake and G.I. Joe have changed drastically from their original design: Strawberry Shortcake is much slimmer and sexier today than she was in the early eighties, and while the original G.I. Joe was, well, an ordinary Joe, today his muscularity exceeds that of a professional bodybuilder. (You can check out these images, and more, on my blog, RachelMarieStone.com.)

One Saturday morning, my mom and I were sitting in a local café, across the street from an outdoor ice-skating rink, watching herds of teenage girls trot around the store in their ski caps and big furry boots which emphasized the skinniness of their pre-pubescent hips and legs in narrow, tight jeans. Only one or two were ever so slightly more rounded in figure; nevertheless, as they gathered up their drinks and settled down in seats near us, we could overhear them talking about their bodies, how much they weighed and calories. "Oh, I weigh 110," said one; "So-and-so at school weighs 125" and so forth. Having wasted years of my own life obsessing over my weight and my body size and every scrap of food I ate (or didn't eat), I wanted to put down my latte and scream at them, "You're perfect as you are! It doesn't matter what you weigh! Please, please, talk about something else!" I didn't do that. But maybe I should have. Their words were dangerous.

I learned the language of dieting and body dissatisfaction from my mom and her friends. When I was about five years old, I wrote a little story called "The Skinny Woman." Depicted in my childish drawing was an extremely tall stick figure wearing high heels. My kindergarten printing explains: "She was pretty. The reason she was so skinny is that she only eats 1 meal a day. The amount she eats is 1 teespon [*sic*]. The moral is: don't eat a lot but don't eat a little bit too!!!" I remember going to Weight Watchers meetings with my mother, seeing her attend church-based diet support groups—FTBT (Free to Be Thin group) was marked for the third Tuesday of each month—and hearing her and her girlfriends endlessly discuss calories and fat and clothing sizes. I'd never been overweight, and I was a particularly skinny child, but I can remember my mom and others sighing over my thinness and saying things like, "Oh, I used to be skinny like that. Just wait until you grow up."

I imagined myself as a self-inflating life vest. One day an invisible valve would release and I'd suddenly inflate and become huge. It wasn't long before I declared war on my imaginary "extra" pounds, refused to eat York Peppermint Patties (my favorite) and took up an exercise program. I bought magazines like *Shape*, wrote down everything I ate and counted calories. I spent hours exercising and hours in front of the mirror thinking hateful things about my body. My parents were aware that something wasn't right, and in part it was their concern and attention that kept me from going further into my disorder. Somehow, my parents could always convince me to join them in eating fried plantains and *sobrebarriga* at the Colombian restaurant I loved or to eat a Belgian waffle with ice cream. I might feel guilty, "fat" and obligated to go for a long jog afterward, but for the time we were at the table, at least, I enjoyed a sweet reprieve from my self-denial.

Others are not so lucky.

THIN (AND EMPTY) NEIGHBORS, SISTERS, DAUGHTERS

Lauren Greenfield's documentary *Thin* introduces several young women who are among the most obvious sufferers in our sick food culture: the anorexic inpatient residents at Florida's Coconut Creek Renfrew Center for eating disorder treatment.

Their skeletal figures are frightening, but their distorted perceptions and preoccupations are more so. They fear losing their skinny figures more than they fear death. Many of them have been more or less forced into treatment by doctors or family members. In reversal of table fellowship's ideal, these very sick women form a community with one another. While the Renfrew staff intend for this to consist of mutual support ("Let's cheer on Polly while she drinks her milkshake!"), the patients, left to themselves, give each other prescription pills on the sly, talk about various strategies for hiding food and compete to be the thinnest.

Yet even these unhealthy relationships are the most significant they've had in years. As the most important thing in their lives is weight loss, they seem able only to understand and be understood by others who live with that all-consuming drive for extreme thinness. The film's companion book highlights a feature of their lives that the film only touches on—that their refusal to eat has made them all so very alone. Consider some of their words:

I just feel like since I was 10, my eating disorder has kept me from life. (Melissa, age 24)[1]

I don't have any connection with anyone. . . . The only thing I've done with my entire life is change my body. (Cara, age 31)[2]

I've distanced myself from friends, family, my parents. . . . It's just a hassle being around people. . . . The eating disorder impacted the relationship with my husband because I felt like he was always in the way. I had missions to accomplish; I had to lose weight. . . . The anorexia is my best friend. (Alisa, age 30)[3]

The book shows their detailed lists and journal ramblings. One attempted suicide after being unable to regurgitate two pieces of pizza; another spent $1,500 monthly on food only to vomit it all up; another writes letters to "Ana"—anorexia personified—longing for the day when she can get out of the treatment center and once again devote herself to worshiping that unholy goddess of thin. Another complains about the weight she's been forced to gain in treatment: "This masterpiece [my body] that I painted, they're just ruining it, and I can't do anything about it."[4]

Around a fifth of anorexics lose their lives to the disease, the deadliest of all mental illnesses. Thirty to 40 percent make a full recovery; the rest cycle in and out of hospitals and treatment programs, perhaps able to hold a job and some relationships, but remain haunted by their disorder, unable to live fully and freely. Inpatient centers like Renfrew currently offer the best mainstream choice for treatment, but relapses are common. Shelly, one of the women in the film, remarked that she wanted to continue being force-fed formula through a stomach tube "because eating is just way too complicated." Her friend Polly noted feeling scared when a cookie she was required to eat tasted good, and talked about how, at thirty years of age, she has no idea how to go food shopping, having never experienced normal desire, pleasure and satisfaction toward food.[5] "Do I *like* cookies now?" she agonizes. Though Shelly, after some relapses, is doing quite well,[6] Polly died two years after the documentary premiered.[7]

In writing about her "real recovery"—as opposed to her "bull$#!+ recovery" (the "recovery" she made at Renfrew and other treatment centers), Shelly tells of the influence of eating with others—a kind of experience that couldn't have taken place in an inpatient treatment setting:

> I surrounded myself with people who have "normal" eating habits. I watched them eat (but not that crazy, obsessive "let me watch people while I don't eat a thing"). I was doing research. I watched them enjoy the food and they didn't feel guilty. I wanted to be like that.

Shelly's family's despair over her illness also cemented in her mind the need to recover fully, and she has done that. Recently Shelly told me that thanks to long walks with her dog, quality family therapy and tae kwon do, she's still in recovery. Surrounding herself with *healthy* eaters proved helpful in a way that focusing on her fears in the company of other ill women at Renfrew couldn't.[8] Alcoholics who are still drinking form communities known as "drinking buddies"; only alcoholics who have stopped drinking can support each other in AA.

When Laura Collins's daughter Olympia became ill with anorexia, Collins and her husband were unsatisfied with their treatment options—they didn't want to send their daughter away to an inpatient facility, and Olympia's counselor seemed to be stirring up mistrust between Olympia and her parents. An outpatient program they tried merely offered Olympia the opportunity to brush up on self-starvation techniques. Collins, a writer, was determined to help her daughter, so she searched the library and the Internet for effective treatment methods, ultimately discovering for herself a lesser-known model: family-based treatment/therapy (FBT), also known as the Maudsley approach. She writes about her family's journey in her 2005 book, *Eating with Your Anorexic.* Pioneered at London's Maudsley Hospital, family-based therapy for eating disorders was inspired by the caring practice of nurses who would sit for hours with anorexic patients, rubbing their backs, speaking soothingly to them and creating an environment in which it was "impossible to not eat." The development of family-based therapy was also motivated by economic reasons: treating eating disorders at home costs far less than treatment at inpatient facilities. Renfrew's inpatient program, for example, costs $1,500 per *day*; their services, categorized as "mental health treatment," are often inadequately covered by insurance plans.

FBT sounds simple enough. Under the guidance of a doctor, a nutritionist and a Maudsley-sympathetic counselor, you sit down for three meals and two snacks a day with your anorexic loved one and *eat with them.* Just as someone with AIDS must take their antiretrovirals and someone with diabetes must take their insulin injections, someone who is starving must eat. An anorexic's medicine is food, and in FBT the family gathers around their frightened, starving loved one to support and encourage them as they take their medicine. Life gets put on hold while the suffering person relearns that most basic of behaviors—*eating.*

For so long, it has been assumed that no one—least of all parents—should *make* anorexics eat. They'll eat when their underlying issues are resolved, it's often said. Following the theories of Hilde Bruch's universally cited *The Golden Cage,*[9] anorexia has been popularly understood to be motivated by issues of control, specifically, by wanting to assert autonomy in the face of parental control or perfectionism. It's frequently said that anorexia is "not about the food" and "not about wanting to be thin"—despite the fact that many, if not most, anorexics do claim to want thinness above all. Alissa says, "This is what I really want. I want to be thin,

and if it takes dying to get there, so be it." Brittany clutches her
fists and wails in a group session, "I just want to be thin! I just
want to be thin!" Shelly admits that although she's got "issues,"
she's not sure *why* she has anorexia. "Maybe I just want to be thin,"
she says.

The reason for "re-feeding" first has to do with the fact that
many of the psychological characteristics of anorexia are identical
with the characteristics of starvation itself.

In an ominously titled mid-1940s study—the "Minnesota Starvation Experiment"—Ancel Keys and his researchers underfed
thirty-six healthy young men for six months, cutting their daily
calories from a healthy 3,200 to 1,560 calories, mostly in the form
of potatoes, rutabagas, turnips and bread. Most lost 25 percent of
their body weight and experienced extreme emotional distress,
including depression, hysteria, compulsive behaviors, preoccupation with food, phobias, aggression and social withdrawal. One
man cut off one of his fingers. After six months of semi-starvation,
the men were returned to normal rations—but it took up to *eight
months* of re-feeding for their psychological profiles to return to
normal.[10] Proponents of FBT point to this study to show that talk
therapy with actively restricting anorexics is more or less a losing
race against death. Turns out counseling works *much* better if you
first bring the patient back from the edge of suicide by starvation.
Counseling an acutely ill anorexic person is not unlike engaging
in post-trauma psychotherapy with a gunshot victim without
stanching the flow of blood and calling in the life-support team.

FBT is powerful. Recovery statistics are cited as close to 90
percent, or more than twice the recovery rate of traditional approaches. In her 2010 memoir *Brave Girl Eating,* Harriet Brown
tells about her daughter Kitty's successful recovery through FBT,
explaining that, like Laura Collins, she was frightened by the *One
Flew Over the Cuckoo's Nest* feel of the residential facilities as well
as the poor recovery rates. It took enormous—though not super-

human—determination and effort, but Brown and her husband rearranged their lives in order to be with Kitty for every meal and every snack of every day. Though she doubted her ability to undertake such a task, she also had that very thing that casts out fear. In her words:

> We have something no one else in the world has: we love Kitty best. No one else in the world can possibly want her to get better as much as we do. No one else loves her as fiercely, as nonjudgmentally, as unconditionally as we do.[11]

In both the Brown and Collins families, meals suddenly *had* to become a priority—both mothers write of putting effort into cooking as never before. Each note that while no one questions the necessity of quitting work to care for a loved one with, say, terminal cancer, committing to long hours at home to feed one's starving child is somehow less understandable. And both speak of the eventual, near-miraculous *enjoyment* that their families discovered in the shared meal. Critics of FBT sometimes complain that the approach makes anorexics dependent on their parents to make them eat. Indeed, Kitty relapsed her first year away from her parents, and Olympia still "looked to [her parents] to support her eating and her choices" one year after beginning her treatment. But what if that theoretical "personal choice" to eat is not a move we're supposed to have to make anyway? As Collins writes:

> For most people in the world, food is not something you make many choices about. Most people get up and eat the same food their ancestors ate. Dietary choices are the luxury—and bane—of modern American life. Perhaps this constant choosing and innovation and individual decision making is really more aberrant than freeing.[12]

Brown also, though she had once struggled with food and body image as most American women do, found herself reacting against aberrant American attitudes toward food, recognizing them finally as insane:

> We . . . have fallen for the notion that food is a regrettable necessity. As if the ideal, the holy grail we are all working toward, is to do without food altogether—and as if we not only should but could attain this state, were we good enough, determined enough, strong enough. As if that's what we should want.[13]

In these stories, the simple act of eating together—with love and with caring, informed support—brings to life people walking toward death.

ALL OF US

In truth, we're all walking toward death—some of us at a brisker pace than others—but sharing meals with others helps all of us come a little bit more alive.

I used to eat a lot of "energy" bars—artificially chocolate-flavored, vitamin-enriched isolated protein chunks that had a chalky chewiness and left a metallic tang on my tongue. They were unsatisfying, but I always wanted more of them. When I ate too many of them at a time, I felt bloated, which made me feel fat, which made me hate myself. Oh, and I always ate them alone. That's more or less how they're designed to be eaten. You don't really say to someone, "Hey, we should get together for some energy bars sometime!" Energy bars are for solitary eating by design.

But a pot of split pea soup—such as Kym and I prepared together one evening—is designed for eating with others. You can thin it with milk and stretch it to feed more people. No one's stomach could possibly expand to hold it all, and if you had to eat it by yourself until it was gone, you'd probably be really tired of it. Soup is community food, and not just because that's what's served at soup kitchens or by the magician in the old tale of "Stone Soup."

My dad had a lot of girlfriends in his youth, and many of them were, well, not thin. But when they went out to eat, they always ordered salads. Dad would think (but not say), *Listen, you don't exactly slide under the door. I'm pretty sure you don't live on salad.* (Maureen, with whom I once waited tables, would roll her eyes when our fuller-figured customers ordered side salads and nothing else. *Darn it, I know you're gonna go home and order a pizza! Just eat a real meal already.*) My dad had the impression that his dates were embarrassed to be seen eating a real meal, that they thought it wasn't feminine, reminiscent of how Scarlett in *Gone with the Wind* was supposed to eat lunch before the barbeque, so everyone would think she has a dainty appetite.

Many people suffer from anorexia's less-glamorized *doppelganger,* compulsive eating disorder, which manifests itself in public salad-eating and private cake-snarfing. (My energy bar binges kind of qualify.) People who restrict their eating try to hide that fact. Those who eat compulsively also do it in secret, because who wants to be seen frantically shoveling in a pint of Ben & Jerry's ice cream with a potato chip chaser? The obesity that tends to result from this eating is itself a mark of shame. People who are heavy sometimes say that they don't like to be seen eating because they're afraid people will think, *You pig! Don't you know that eating is what's making you fat?* This despite several important but ignored facts: not everyone who is obese is unhealthy, not everyone who is obese has binge eating disorder and not everyone who binges uncontrollably ends up obese. It's not possible to judge based on people's appearances, but I think it's safe to say that doing most of our eating *with others,* well, is safest.

But the first time my dad took out my mom, he was charmed: she ordered a cheeseburger platter and a milkshake, and not only did she eat heartily, she finished her fries and helped herself companionably to a few of his. She didn't exactly "slide under the door,"

either, and he admired her unembarrassed, *honest* enjoyment of
food—a rare thing, in his experience. He loved her for it.

> She could feel hunger, and she could satisfy it. It wasn't, as she feared,
> that once she conceded hunger, that desire would completely over-
> whelm her and she would eat everything in sight. Quite the opposite.
> Hunger had limits, and once she paid attention, they were easy to find.
> As she practiced, she learned that all desires had limits and even
> orders. They were all essentially "good," but not every one had to be
> satisfied at exactly the same moment. She could put them in proper
> contexts—choose to satisfy one desire now or put off another for a
> better moment. To name and to satisfy one's desires was not, contrary
> to what she had long believed, to be at the mercy of selfishness and
> sin. On the contrary, naming and satisfying took her step-by-step onto
> a path toward life and goodness.
> —Amy Frykholm, *See Me Naked*

If I were to put out my hands to receive Communion only to
have the priest snarl, "You don't deserve any, you dirty sinner! I
heard you screaming at your kids before you came into church!" I
would leave and never come back. Communion is grace, and grace
doesn't come to me because I deserve it. But giving ourselves grace
isn't easy, and it's not easy to give it to others either. Yet eating
with others can be a means of grace, a grace that can keep all our
eating graces, to paraphrase the poet Gerard Manley Hopkins.[14]

It's no accident that praying before eating is often called "saying
grace." It's not just that we are thanking God for the food, though
we're doing that. We are also making a point of noticing that our
food comes from God. The words we use to talk about food and
bodies matter, as well, because they nourish and shape and feed
us—or poison, warp and starve us—every bit as much as food does.
Who can eat gratefully and joyfully while thinking, *I'm an ugly pig*

who doesn't deserve to eat? I couldn't. Who can eat with real pleasure when the table talk centers on dimply thighs, flabby bellies, calories, cholesterol and what's "healthy" or "unhealthy"? No one can, and such talk actually fuels disorder in the form of *over*eating at least as much as it fuels disorder in the form of *under*eating.

The psychology researcher Eric Stice discovered that women and girls who spent three hours a week verbally affirming healthy attitudes toward their bodies and tried, as much as possible, to avoid "fat talk," were much less likely to develop eating disorders.[15] Our bodies, God's masterpieces, deserve grace and care. I would never call my children's paintings or Play-Doh sculptures or Lego creations ugly. God sees my permanent under-eye circles and long graceful fingers and shiny scars and flat feet and glossy hair and calls it *all* good, because he made it all, and because he let himself be broken to heal what brokenness is in me. And in you too.

Anne Lamott tells a story of going shopping with her best friend, Pammy, who was weak from chemo and a month from death. Anne tried on a tight lavender dress—she wanted to impress her boyfriend—and asked Pammy if she thought the dress made her hips look big. Gently, Pammy said, "Anne, you don't have that kind of time."[16] A dying person knows that there just isn't time in life to spend not *living*, and obsessing about hips (or lips or tummies) isn't really living. ("Heaven," said Bette Midler, "would be a place where people would stop talking about their weight and what they look like.")[17] I don't have time for chalky energy bars snarfed in solitude, or for wondering whether I "deserve" to eat lunch. What we all have time for, what we all deserve, is a seat at the table, eating in the company of people who give us grace.

I think of the stories of Olympia, Kitty and the women at the Renfrew Centers as coal-mine canary stories. Most of us won't get clinically diagnosable forms of eating disorders, but we'll get the bite-sized version that gets hold of us best when we're just too alone. North American food culture has strayed far from the communal table and its traditions. Our freedom to eat whatever, whenever, however (it used to be considered rude to eat between meals or alone) has scared us alternately into secretive snarfing or starving. We need to be able to eat French fries off each other's plates and love each other more, not less, because of it. We need other people to love us back to joy, and other people need us to do likewise for them—each of us priests and each of us communicants, saying without words and with each bite: "The body of Christ broken for you—the bread of heaven; the blood of Christ shed for you—the cup of salvation."

PRAYERS BEFORE EATING

For each new morning with its light,
For rest and shelter of the night,
For health and food,
For love and friends,
For everything Thy goodness sends.
Attributed to Ralph Waldo Emerson (1803-1882)

Be present at our table, Lord,
Be here and everywhere adored.
Thy creatures bless and grant that we
May feast in paradise with Thee. Amen.

We thank you, our God,
for every earthly good:
for life and health and family,
and for our daily food.
Amen.

RECIPES

Curried Red Lentil Soup
It sounds kind of unappetizing to say so, but this is a great clean-

out-the-fridge soup. (Be judicious concerning food safety rules, please!) Lots of different kinds of veggies—and even fruits— blend in wonderfully.

Chop these into small dice, and don't bother to peel first—just scrub, then chop.

1 large yellow onion
4 stalks celery
8 carrots
4 potatoes
4 apples

Other things: chopped green beans, leftover mashed potatoes, etc. (optional)

In a large soup pot, heat **4 tablespoons olive oil** until shiny. Add **4 cloves garlic, minced finely,** and a **peeled, grated, 1-inch piece of ginger.** Cook several minutes, until fragrant, and add the onion. Cook 10 minutes, and add the rest of the veggies, stirring constantly. Cook for 20 minutes or so, adding more oil if necessary, until the mixture is highly fragrant and the carrots and apples begin to caramelize. Sprinkle **1 or 2 teaspoons curry spices** over, and continue stirring for 1 minute. Pour over **4 cups vegetable stock** (or water, in a pinch) and scrape the bottom and sides of the pot vigorously, releasing all the lovely browned bits. Add **1 can diced tomatoes (or 1 1/2 cups chopped fresh tomatoes)** and **1 cup washed, presoaked and drained red lentils.** If it looks like it needs more liquid, add a bit more water. Allow the soup to simmer, covered, for 45 minutes; then taste and adjust seasonings, adding **salt** and **pepper,** or a bit more **curry** (mixed with cold water first), if needed, and the **juice from 1 lemon.** Serve with plain full-fat yogurt and unsweetened dried coconut as toppings, and with bread—especially the no-knead bread—for dipping.

Black Bean & Corn Quinoa

This is such a quick and easy meal. It's delicious topped with sour cream, salsa and black olives, and scooped up with tortilla chips. You can even roll it up in tortillas and eat it like a burrito. However, it's great all on its own, too, drizzled with a bit of lime juice.

Heat a large skillet with a lid until a drop of water sizzles. Add ¼ cup olive oil and heat until shimmering. Add 2 large yellow onions, chopped, and 1 tablespoon minced garlic. Cook, stirring frequently, until soft and brown, about 10 minutes. Sprinkle with 1 teaspoon dried oregano, 1/2 teaspoon cumin, 1 teaspoon paprika, and stir. Pour in 1 1/2 cup rinsed and drained quinoa and salt and pepper, stirring constantly for 5 minutes, or until quinoa looks a bit browned. Add 1 can (or cooked equivalent) black beans, drained, 1 cup frozen corn kernels and 3 cups vegetable stock or water. Bring to a boil, reduce heat to low, stir and cover for 20 minutes. Fluff the quinoa kernels lightly with a fork when they are finished and serve.

• •

POINTS FOR ACTION

- Make your house, and especially your table, a "fat talk"–free zone.

- Openly critique unrealistic images of bodies you see in magazines and on television.

- If you are a parent, and you have a poor self-image or disordered attitudes and behaviors toward eating, it is worth considering working through those for your sake as well as those of your children. Such attitudes and behaviors are often passed on from parent to child.

- Consciously and attentively thank God for your food, and praise God for the beauty and grace of human bodies.

- An alternative to body hatred might be noticing what works well in your body and giving thanks for it, or taking time to nourish and care for your body in a new way, by taking a walk or putting lotion on your dry skin, even and especially on the parts (thighs? stomach?) that you tend not to like.

• You might also consider volunteering in a food-related ministry. It could be as simple as bringing a meal or special snack to someone who is elderly or ill. Ministering to others with food can be re-orienting.

5

Sustainable Eating

WISE CHOICES IN
STEWARDING THE LAND

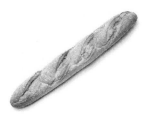

Years ago my husband and I, along with some friends, backpacked for nine days in the Beartooth Wilderness in Montana, the state where Tim grew up. To get to the chilly, shimmering trio of related lakes near which we made camp,[1] we crossed boulder fields and rivers and grassy hillsides so steep we had to use our hands to keep from falling. After we camped by the lake, we saw no one from outside our group for the entire time. From our base camp, we embarked on various day hikes, one time reaching the summit of an 11,000-foot peak. Up there no trees can grow, and there is a minimum of brush.

On the way to the peak, we encountered a family of mountain goats. The gentle, curious creatures fearlessly gathered around Tim for a good look, sniffing at his pack and giving him their best goatly welcome. As I watched them make their way up a cliff face that I couldn't have scaled on my best day, I shivered with a feeling that was pleasant despite being surprisingly like sadness or loneliness, a feeling that came again at the summit, where I found to my delight tiny flowers growing almost flat against the rocky surface.

That feeling of lonely sadness was pierced by a sudden, sharp sense of God's own pleasure and delight in these wild things. I don't think that I had ever before been so far into the wilderness, beyond all that, as Gerard Manley Hopkins wrote, "wears man's smudge and shares man's smell,"[2] so far away from all that could be bought and sold or advertised or made useful. The goats were doing well up there above the tree line—there were babies in their tribe, evidence of their flourishing—with no help from any person at all. They would not become meat for anyone's plate any more than the flowers would be picked for someone's table. Even remembering our brief and improbable encounter brings me joy and moves me to worship the God of wild things, and to recall that the earth is not, finally, mine.

God gives humans "dominion" over the earth and its creatures as a *blessing* in Genesis 1:28: "Be fruitful and multiply, and fill the earth and subdue it; and have dominion over the fish of the sea and over the birds of the air and over every living thing that moves upon the earth." This passage has often served as the basis for a Christian understanding of what is often called "stewardship." Even where writers have sought to avoid using this verse as a license for exploitation, they've still taken it to imply that humans stand *above* the rest of creation and that, because of this, we're free to make whatever use of the earth we wish. Nancy Pearcey, among others, finds in this verse the motive and justification for modern science and technology.[3]

I learned to be suspicious of "environmentalism" from my Christian curriculum materials and the children's version of *World* magazine, while my wise grandmother kept me subscribed to *National Geographic Kids.* I was drawn to stories of ecological crises and species extinction and the efforts of ordinary children to make a difference in the health of the planet, but I always suspected, guiltily, that my concern for animals or for the health of the rain-forests might in fact constitute "exchang[ing] the truth about God for a lie and worship[ing] and serv[ing] the creature rather than the Creator" (Rom 1:25). Even as I write, there are "Worship the Creator, not the Creation" and other such Facebook groups denying that humans pose any threat to the earth's well-being while asserting that caring for creation constitutes nature worship. But, encouragingly, many Christians have begun to take what's frequently called "creation care" seriously, rediscovering what has in fact been a rich Christian tradition.

Perhaps, as Bill McKibben suggests, the present ecological crisis has opened our eyes to the truth that God cares very deeply about the earth; that the Scripture's agricultural background is more than just *background* to the drama between God and people, and is in fact a valid and applicable concern in itself.[4] A number of books—among them, *Making Peace with the Land, Keeping God's Earth, Green Like God* and *The Bible and Ecology*—have called Christians to reconsider their role within the created order and to work for a kind of reconciliation with the earth and our co-creatures, to help work toward the ideal of the peaceable kingdom where the "wolf shall live with the lamb, the leopard shall lie down with the kid, the calf and the lion and the fatling together, and a little child shall lead them" (Is 11:6).

As the novelist and essayist Marilynne Robinson writes, "Our doings on this planet [are] wildly exceptional, whatever else may be said about them."[5] It's true: human beings, and their doings, are nothing short of astonishing—just a little lower than the angels. Yet we are also envisioned in Scripture as *co-creatures* within the created realm—members in the community of creation. In all of life, we are called to serve and protect the earth in ways that allow for human flourishing while also guarding the well-being of the earth and the life on it—both animal and vegetable, remembering that first and foremost the earth and everything in it belongs to

God. As Robinson writes elsewhere, "The laws of Moses assume that the land is *God's;* that the Hebrews are strangers and sojourners there who cannot really own it but who enjoy it at God's pleasure (Leviticus 25:23)."[6]

BROTHERS AND SISTERS WITH CREATION

There's a Christmas song that begins, "Jesus our brother, strong and good / Was humbly born in a stable rude / And the friendly beasts around him stood." In the following verses, the various animals traditionally imagined in Jesus' stable tell about "the gifts they gave Emmanuel." For example: "I, said the donkey, shaggy and brown / I carried his mother up hill and down / I carried her safely to Bethlehem town."[7] It's a quirky song, but I love its earthiness; I love imagining animals humbly serving the Firstborn of Creation in their simple way. I've never heard it sung in church; maybe it just feels too weird for people to sing about Jesus in the persona of a nonhuman creature.[8] Yet the Bible doesn't share our reluctance to put words of praise into the mouths of both animals *and* inanimate creation:

> Praise the LORD from the earth,
>   you sea monsters and all deeps,
> fire and hail, snow and frost,
>   stormy wind fulfilling his command!
>
> Mountains and all hills,
>   fruit trees and all cedars!
> Wild animals and all cattle,
>   creeping things and flying birds!
>
> Kings of the earth and all peoples,
>   princes and all rulers of the earth!
> Young men and women alike,
>   old and young together!

Let them praise the name of the LORD,
    for his name alone is exalted;
    his glory is above earth and heaven. (Ps 148:7-13)

I love that "all peoples"—even kings, princes and rulers—are
grouped together with sea creatures, elements of weather, animals,
birds and plants in a chorus of praise to the Lord. Those goats and
flowers in the Montana mountains sang their songs of praise just by
being there. Yet for many, it's uncomfortable to think of people as
lowly co-creatures along with the animals. St. Francis, a notable
exception in Christian history, called all animals "brother" and
"sister" and referred to his own body as "Brother Ass." But Francis's
comfort with his own "creatureliness" is by no means common.[9]
Strange as it may seem, the Bible tends to envision us similarly—as
creatures dwelling in God's creation, lower than God, higher than
animals, but ultimately created beings.[10] While Christian thinking
about humanity's relationship to the environment has frequently
overemphasized Genesis 1, looking at the biblical wisdom more
broadly invites us to think of ourselves as members within the community of creation, not sovereigns over it.[11]

As an antidote to human arrogance, both Bill McKibben[12] and
Richard Bauckham point to the book of Job, especially to chapters
38–39, where God answers Job out of the whirlwind to tell him to
hush it: he has no idea how the universe or anything in it works.
Throughout, it's clear that God, and God alone, can hold back the
seas, command the weather, turn the seasons and know intimately
the lives of all wild creatures. He questions Job repeatedly, saying
to him, "Explain these mysteries to me, if you're so smart!" Of
course, Job has nothing to say except:

    See, I am of small account; what shall I answer you?
        I lay my hand on my mouth.
    I have spoken once, and I will not answer;
        twice, but will proceed no further. (Job 40:3-5)

Tasting the "strong medicine"[13] of God's words, Job finds he has nothing to say.

We *are* different from the animals; our God-given role in creation is special. But it's just that—a *role*. Old Testament scholar Daniel Block suggests that we have frequently misconstrued the "image of God" to mean that our ontology—that is, the nature of our being—is qualitatively different from that of the animals. Rather, he says, we are "one with land animals, who were also created on day 6." He argues that the image of God is really more about *function* than about *substance*—more about our *role* within creation than a special *quality* of our being. And our role is to "serve" and "guard" the rest of creation. These words in Hebrew, explains Block, rather than asserting our supremacy over nature, instead demand that we "expend [our] efforts in the interests of and for the well-being of the object" of our service and guardianship. In the world, then, we serve as God's deputies and representatives. In that role, we're called to recognize the sacramentality of all life.[14] To our fellow creatures—and even to inanimate creation—we are *in loco Dei*—in the place of God.

Our present ecological crises—the endless landfills, the smog-belching cars and factories, the changes in weather patterns, the depletion of soil fertility and extinction of species—demonstrate our shortcomings in this high calling, which is the nice way of saying that the state of creation disgraces us. "I think we all know," writes Marilynne Robinson, "that the earth might be reaching the end of its tolerance for our presumptions."[15]

Without evading the guilt that is surely ours for our complicity in the many destructive abuses inflicted on the earth and our fellow creatures, it is also true that the creation "has been groaning in labor pains" (Rom 8:22)—that all is not as it ought to be on earth, and that we can't fix it on our own. God's "eco-topian" ideal—where the "cow and the bear shall graze . . . and the lion shall eat straw like the ox" (Is 11:7)—is obviously not a present reality. The picture of Eden's garden is one of peaceful, harmonious communion existing between animals and people, with soil easily and happily yielding food for all. *This* was—and is—God's intention. The Bible's vision of the new creation involves the *entire* earth in the redemption story, picturing the new creation as a new Eden—except that it will then fill all the earth. Living between Eden and the new creation, we can neither return to the garden nor bring about the New Jerusalem by our own efforts. We're *no longer* there, and we're *not yet* there.

While the new creation will involve "radical transformation," it will *not* entail a wholesale replacement of this present earth.[16] In conquering death and rising from the grave, Jesus began God's new creation; as Jesus' followers, we live in the days of the new creation—and so any work we do in him will last. Our efforts to renew God's beloved creation are *not* akin to "oiling the wheels of a machine that's about to roll over a cliff," "restoring a great painting that's shortly going to be thrown on the fire" or "planting roses in a garden that's about to be dug up for a building site." Instead, in taking seriously our responsibility to "serve" and "guard" creation, we are, "strange though it may seem, almost as hard to believe as the resurrection itself—accomplishing something that will become . . . part of God's new world."[17]

PEACEFUL FARMING

What does it look like to raise food in light of our role as God's ministers for creation care? Food production contributes enormously to our present environmental crises. Right behind automobiles, producing food consumes more oil than any other sector of the American economy.[18] Whereas a hundred years ago, virtually all food was what we'd now consider "organic" and "local," and more than half of Americans lived on farms, today just one percent live on farms.[19] While organic, local foods are enjoying huge growth, conventionally produced food is by far the norm and is generally cheaper (in sticker price only) than organic and local alternatives. The growing techniques that are called "conventional" use chemicals that are dangerous to the degree that farm workers have demonstrably higher rates of cancer, respiratory diseases and other ailments associated with the poisons they must use on the food we eat.[20]

Animal feeding practices, too, have changed drastically in the past century. Cattle for beef once lived on land largely unsuited for row-crops—such as the ranch my father-in-law grew up on. Being ruminants, cows are great at converting plants unsuitable for human consumption—grass—into food—meat. Today, though, it's the rare and lucky cow that gets to live and die eating grass—the vast majority of them live in crowded, filthy, concentrated animal-feeding operations (CAFOs) eating genetically modified corn mixed with antibiotics and other questionable substances, emitting methane gases and filling giant "lagoons" with their excrement, which in turn create runoff that seriously pollutes the water around them—because it's cheaper (again, in supermarket price only) to raise beef this way.

How did we get to this place, and is there any hope of getting back to a system of food production that allows for creation—and for us within creation—to flourish?

Journalist Michael Pollan tells the story of the German Jewish chemist Fritz Haber, a man few of us have heard of, though he (somewhat ironically) won the Nobel Prize in 1918 for "improving the standards of agriculture and the well-being of mankind" by creating the first artificial process for "fixing" nitrogen. All life depends on nitrogen—it is the "building block from which nature assembles amino acids, proteins and nucleic acid"—but the earth's supply of usable nitrogen is limited. Haber was the first to figure out how to take atoms of nitrogen from the atmosphere and combine them into useful molecules, and it won him the Nobel Prize. Millions of people exist on earth today because of him.

Fixing nitrogen synthetically led to the development of chemical fertilizers that greatly increased crop yields and probably saved China from famine in the 1970s.

But fixing nitrogen by Haber's process involves an enormous amount of fossil fuel, and it also made industrial-scale agriculture possible. Chemical fertilizers also have some serious drawbacks, not least "blue baby" syndrome and nitrogen-caused "dead zones" in bodies of water. Haber's own life reflected his work; both embody "the paradoxes of science, the double edge to our manipulations of nature, the good and evil that can flow not only from the same man but from the same knowledge." During World War I, he lent his genius to the German war effort, using synthetic nitrate to make bombs. He also helped develop poison gases, including, in sick irony, Zyklon B, the gas used in Nazi concentration camps. His wife took her own life using his pistol, disgusted at his part in the war, and he died alone in a hotel room, a broken man.[21]

Haber's story is at once an illustration of the incredible capacities of human beings—who would have thought it was possible for a human to fix nitrogen?—as well as our frailties. Synthetic nitrogen fertilizers fed a lot of people, yes, but also made it possible to drop bombs on a lot of people. Synthetic insecticides and herbicides, which derived from the poison gases of World War II, have helped control pest and weed problems and made high yields of corn possible, but that very abundance has led to another kind of trouble.

One of the reasons that the high yield of corn is such a problem is that it is not really food; it's a raw material for processing into anything and everything from ethanol to steak (by using CAFO-imprisoned cows as corn-converting machines) to Twizzlers. What looks like diversity in the supermarket is in fact clever engineering that makes endless varieties of corn-based products appear to be different foods. This is economically advantageous for the handful of companies that profit from the heavily tax-subsidized crops. And the corn we eat in myriad ways isn't the old-fashioned stuff that

Squanto taught the Pilgrims to cultivate either. Some estimates suggest that nearly 90 percent of all corn grown in the United States is one of several patented, genetically engineered varieties.[22]

PLEASE, NO GMO

What's most striking about GMOs (genetically modified organisms) and the companies that produce them is that they're patented life. Most seed varieties are now under patent by private corporations, in effect *owned* by them—as if anyone could *really* own the life that only God can create.[23] Certain patented seeds are sold with the stipulation that farmers may not save seed for next year's planting; they must buy more seeds from the company. Several strains have been altered genetically to contain a "suicide gene" that makes the seeds produced by the next generation sterile, ending that millennia-long practice of saving seeds and requiring the farmer to be dependent on the seed company for as long as he wishes to plant: planned obsolescence in biological life. Worse, GMO seeds spread, as seeds do, to fields where they are decidedly unwanted.[24]

Agribusiness corporations have also developed seed products that they would have us believe will save the world. Golden rice, for example, is a variety of rice genetically modified to contain vitamin A. Some believe that its tiny yellow grains may hold the potential to prevent the blindness that comes from severe vitamin A deficiency; many others feel that Golden rice could potentially exacerbate malnutrition by creating dependence on a single industrial crop, rather than solving malnutrition the old fashioned way—by introducing other foods that compose a balanced diet.[25] And because vitamin A is fat-soluble, Golden rice must be eaten with adequate dietary fat to be properly absorbed—but since its target consumers often lack this too, the benefit of this rice would effectively be nil.

Knowing that the use of GMO seeds creates dependence,

Haitian officials refused to use GMO seeds that had been donated by Monsanto in the aftermath of their tragic earthquake.[26] If you convince farmers that food can't be grown without special seed, without pesticides, herbicides and chemical fertilizers, you can make them dependent on your products for life—or at least until their money runs out. One reason that you'll sometimes hear representatives of agribusiness dismissing organic agriculture as nice but impractical for feeding a hungry planet is that there really isn't a whole lot of money to be made from things like poop, sunshine, crop rotation, composting, biodynamic planting and mulching. But natural ways of controlling pests and weeds and enriching the soil are not only cheaper and thus more accessible to people in the Third World, they are healthier and *more productive* too.[27]

Some will argue that GMOs are simply akin to traditional plant breeding. This sounds comforting but isn't really so. Traditional breeding is a wonder; it's what allowed corn to go from a wild weed with very small kernels of grain to the plump, yellow delicious grain that we know today. As Evelyn Bloch-Dano shows eloquently in her fascinating book *Vegetables: A Biography,* the movement—coaxed along by people—of thistle to artichoke is an important cultural artifact; it's what distinguishes people from donkeys. In fact, almost everything we eat comes to us through hundreds and thousands of years of intentional and accidental domestication. But there's no natural way for a *Bacillus thuringiensis* (Bt) toxin to make it into the genes of corn, no way that genes from a fish could become part of a tomato.

Because of the lack of transparency and accountability on the part of the corporations that control GM production,[28] there's simply no way of knowing what long-term effects genetic modification of seeds might end up having on us, on animals and on the earth. Will the built-in toxins in Bt corn eventually prove toxic to people and animals that eat it? Will GM foods create new food allergies, as some theorize they already have?[29] However marvelous our science—and it *is* marvelous—we must not forget that at the kernel of life there is still a mystery and that, ultimately, it's God's mystery, not ours.

WE DIDN'T CREATE IT; WE DON'T KNOW WHAT IT'S FOR

The other problem stemming from our corn-based agriculture is the frightening loss of diversity in plant life, which, in turn, dangerously and irreparably depletes the soil. Soil depletion is serious business indeed. Bodies are nourished indirectly from the soil; poor soil health means poor health for everyone and everything. Not only is corn used in more places and for more purposes than ever before, but the demands of a highly centralized, homogenized system—a system which, like McDonald's, envisions "one taste worldwide,"[30] have edged out variety in the plant kingdom.

To serve the needs of the fast-food industry, the most-grown variety of potato in the US is by far the familiarly brown-skinned, white-fleshed Russet Burbank, though at the turn of the twentieth century there were thousands of varieties of potatoes grown in the US.[31] (Last year, my family dug up some lawn and planted purple potatoes, just to shake things up. They were beautiful and delicious, but my oldest son wouldn't touch them.) Because crops can be grown most efficiently—planted and harvested by machine on a giant scale—when they are planted in monoculture (that is, huge farms planted with just one kind of seed), this is the way much of our food is produced.

The philosophy of "get big or get out," promoted first during the Eisenhower administration[32] and then again by Earl Butz, secretary of agriculture under former presidents Nixon and Ford, demands huge monocultures and also depends on a huge supply of fossil fuel. Before fossil fuel was available, farmers relied on crop diversity (and homely things like manure) to replenish the soil and to combat pests. Not only is the use of fossil fuel demonstrably unsustainable, the loss of diversity in the fields is bad for human beings and for the earth. Soil forced to produce endless monocultures of corn grows depleted and useless, and that's something none of us can afford to have happen—not the plants, not the animals, not the atmosphere and not us. We're omnivores—we *need* diversity in the fields and in our diets.[33]

True tales warning against the danger of monocultures abound and include the story of the Irish potato famine. In the nineteenth century Irish people, especially the poor, were dependent on large monocultures of potatoes for their food. Cheaper to produce than the former mixed agriculture based on grains and livestock, potatoes were easy to grow and easy to eat, and they became the dietary staple for many Irish. Unfortunately, because monoculture enables the rapid spread of diseases, a microorganism spread quickly throughout Ireland in 1845, blighting the potato harvest that year and for several years following. Out of a population of seven million, one million died and two million emigrated—including some of my ancestors.[34] Given what we've already looked at with respect to our corn-based agriculture, just imagine—what would happen if a *corn* blight were to take hold? Perhaps biodiversity can't prevent famine, but it may be our best hope for doing so.

God values biodiversity as something to be treasured and guarded for its own sake. The Bible, says Block, "place[s] a high stock in . . . biological diversity in general."[35] The early chapters of Genesis indicate God's delight in the variety of what he has made. Psalm 148, which we looked at earlier, seems also to delight in the multitude of varied creatures—animate as well as inanimate—all praising their Creator in concert. Though the biblical writers did not know that biodiversity is key to pest management—monocultures being much more vulnerable to pests than are biologically diverse farms—biodiversity is valued because the millions upon millions of species on earth together form "harmony in the cosmic symphony of praise to God."[36]

I think the words of *another* Nobel laureate, Professor Wangari Maathai, a Kenyan woman, are especially appropriate and wise:

The whole planet earth is a system, and we human species are only part—a very small part—of that system. There are literally millions of species out there. We may not know them, we may not know their value, but we want to conserve them. . . . Don't worry if you don't know what good they are for. You didn't create it, so you don't know what it is for. Just let it be, because who knows: someday down the road, our future generations might find that they can survive because of that aspect of biodiversity.[37]

Professor Maathai was honored with the Nobel Peace Prize for pioneering the Green Belt Movement, a grassroots project among Kenyan women to plant and sustain millions of trees. She's also a Christian. Some were critical of the Nobel committee's decision— how does a massive movement to plant trees contribute to world peace? As Maathai explains in her memoir, *Unbowed*, her tree-planting movement sought to repair the terrible deforestation wrought by the British, who, in colonizing Kenya, "clearcut indigenous forests and replaced them with monoculture plantations of pines and eucalyptus."[38] Lack of firewood needed for cooking, the drying of rivers and creeping desertification all contribute to desperation in Kenya's poorest and most vulnerable people, and the desperation of poverty all too often and easily turns to violence. Planting trees, she explains, fosters peace while caring for people and healing the planet. Saving species is important because it's a way of loving other people, loving God and caring for God's beloved creation. Eating a wide variety of foods is one way of participating in preserving biodiversity.[39] Seeking out food that didn't begin its life as processed corn is a good first step. Planting a garden is another.

WHAT ABOUT ANIMALS?

On the bulletin board in the cafeteria of my conservative Christian

college, someone posted a note asking for more vegetarian options, to which someone replied with scrawl, "God wants you to
eat meat! See Genesis 9!"

Genesis 9, an echo of the original creation blessing in Genesis
1, is often taken as proof positive that God intends for people to
eat meat:

> God blessed Noah and his sons and said to them, "Be fruitful
> and multiply, and fill the earth. The fear and dread of you
> shall rest on every animal of the earth, and on every bird of
> the air, on everything that creeps on the ground, and on all
> the fish of the sea; into your hand they are delivered. Every
> moving thing that lives shall be food for you; and just as I
> gave you the green plants, I give you everything." (Gen 9:1-3)

Yet, this permission to eat meat is a concession, rather than God's
original ideal for creation, which appears wholly nonviolent—all
animals were vegetarian as well, as they will be again in the new
creation. This seems largely uncontroversial: God's ideal is a
peaceful world without violence or death. Shedding blood—
whether human or animal—is always treated with absolute seri-
ousness within Scripture. Eating meat may be permitted, but it's
not pictured in Scripture as God's ideal—either in Eden or in the
new Jerusalem.[40]

On this basis, some Christians (Stephen Webb is a notable
example) insist that the Bible suggests vegetarianism as an
ideal for Christians today. While not to be legislated, he says,
it's to be commended.[41] However, throughout his book, Webb
seems to confuse the biblical ideal of vegetarianism with issues
surrounding how animals are raised in our contemporary
context. Without question, in the United States, the majority of
animals destined for the dinner table are raised in a way that is
degrading, shameful and grievous to God. Numerous books,
articles and documentaries have shed light on this subject, so

I'll be brief in recounting the disgraceful realities.[42]

Animals raised for food in this country are systematically and intentionally tormented, brutalized and exploited in ways that are unlike anything that has ever been done before. They are treated as meat, egg and milk machines, pumped full of hormones and antibiotics, sometimes starved, sometimes force-fed and killed in cruel ways at very early ages—because they're so sick that they would die soon anyway. This system—made possible by the afore-mentioned huge, cheap supply of corn, which is used as feed—contributes enormously to the befouling of the environment and poses real threat to human health for numerous reasons, not least the proliferation of antibiotic-resistant microbes and the development of dangerous strains of E. coli (like O157:H7), to say nothing of BSE, better known as "mad cow disease." Over the last sixty years, meat consumption in the United States has increased by nearly 78 pounds per person per year.[43] Yet though it costs just a few dollars per pound in the supermarket, it is anything but cheap.

Nowhere does the Bible regard animals as objects for human use; rather, as Richard Bauckham points out, the Bible everywhere regards them as subjects of their own lives.[44] The model of a shepherd caring for his sheep is the biblical ideal: a relationship of caring responsibility. The prohibition following God's permission for eating meat begins to hint at this: "You shall not eat flesh with its life, that is, its blood" (Gen 9:4). Block understands this ordinance as one that "forces hunters to identify with the creatures by touching them and personally bearing responsibility for their deaths."[45] Block and Bauckham each point to numerous passages in Scripture that encourage compassionate and caring animal husbandry—passages requiring that animals are given rest (e.g., Deut 5:14), that lost animals are returned (Deut 22:1-3), and that over-burdened animals are relieved and allowed to rest (Ex 23:12). Perhaps most succinct—and, in our present context, convicting—is Proverbs 12:10:

The righteous know the needs of their animals,
     but the mercy of the wicked is cruel.[46]

Block isn't too forceful in pointing to this depressing passage
in Hosea as a word of rebuke to us, who may spend billions annually to feed our pets but are largely oblivious to the suffering of
animals "whose voice is not heard by those whom God has placed
in charge."[47]

The LORD has an indictment against the inhabitants
     of the land.
There is no faithfulness or loyalty,
     and no knowledge of God in the land.
Swearing, lying, and murder,
     and stealing and adultery break out;
     bloodshed follows bloodshed.
Therefore the land mourns,
     and all who live in it languish;
together with the wild animals
     and the birds of the air,
     and even the fish of the sea are perishing. (Hos 4:1-3)

We *don't* have any right to raise and slaughter animals as we
currently do in this country. Many people will, on this basis,
follow a vegetarian (or vegan) diet. My family ate vegetarian for
some time because we couldn't find free-range meat. But eventually we decided to seek out the small farmers who raise and
slaughter animals in ways that are sustainable and respectful,
like Joel Salatin. Paying the *true* cost of quality meat means for
many of us that we'll eat far less of it, which is a good thing for
our well-being and that of the planet. (Plus, free-range meat is
rich in the kinds of fats that are understood to be *good* for
us, whereas feedlot meat—fed on corn—is rich in the fats that
aren't so good, especially in excess.) Further, we have chosen, for
the most part, to eat what is served to us by other people, feeling

that in a choice between offending our host and eating food that doesn't reflect our values, love for our (human) neighbor takes priority.

While meat eating is undoubtedly a concession, and while the way animals are raised for food is unacceptable for so many reasons, the truth is that most people eat meat and don't plan to stop anytime soon. The reasons for eating less meat are pretty compelling, but there are also good reasons to continue to eat meat, doing so thoughtfully rather than mindlessly.

While it's true the biblical vision of eating in the nonviolent new creation (as in Eden) doesn't involve animal slaughter, it also doesn't seem to involve much agriculture at all. Adam and Eve aren't fussing over their orchard; they're picking and eating what God appears to have already tended to. In both places, God does all the feeding. In both places, the earth spontaneously yields all kinds of plants that are good for food. We're familiar with what Eden looked like in that respect, and the tree of life in Revelation 22 echoes Eden, but even better—it yields twelve kinds of fruit.

In the new creation, something radically different—a new creative work on God's part—will take place. Right now, it's biologically impossible for a lion (or, for that matter, a house cat) to be a vegetarian. For "true shalom [to] reign over all," God will do something entirely new.[48] But in this present world, carnivorous animals are part of the ecosystem. Trying to change this would be impossible and, possibly, dangerous. While some argue that we, unlike animals, can choose a vegetarian diet, this is true only of some—certainly not of all—people in the world. Many—even those who were until a few years ago middle class—don't have the luxury of being choosy about their food. During my parents' lean young-family years, our protein came from Spam and government cheese because that's what they could afford, and that's what was given to them in the bags of groceries they gratefully accepted from others. In many places people have no access to supplies of protein and fat—and in the case of Inuit people, calories—that do not come from the bodies of dead animals.

Choosing not to eat animals that have been tortured is, I think, a separate question from eating animals that have been treated with respect and allowed to live their natural lives as God intended. Eating that kind of meat—from animals that have been well cared for—can actually help change animal agriculture for the better. Barbara Kingsolver and Joel Salatin point to humane, well-tended farms whose respectful treatment of animals helped convince a number of vegans to diversify their diets so as to be able to support farmers who raise and slaughter animals with mercy and reverence. (You can visit LocalHarvest .org to find humanely raised meat near you; they ship on dry ice.)

Eliminating animals from human diets isn't always the sustainable choice for the simple reason that animals are essential on a biodynamic farm. To put it in terms that my children find hilarious: their poop, so problematic when they live on CAFOs, replenishes the soil beautifully. Animals living on pasture also make it possible to turn grass or other inedible vegetation into nutritious milk, meat and eggs. In many places, irrigation or soil conditions make growing lots of vegetables impossible, but hardy goats and other ruminants can live by eating whatever growing things they come across, and, in turn, they feed the people who care for them. So having an animal to use for milk, eggs and, eventually, meat greatly improves both the lives of the people and the health of the soil, and thus the health of the ecosystem. That's why organizations like Heifer International, which do so much to return dignity and beauty to the lives of the poorest people on the planet, focus on teaching responsible animal husbandry.

Eating meat can be a part of a compassionate, humane and joyful relationship with food, but most of us would do well to eat less of it and to purchase, when we can, sustainably and humanely produced meat, dairy and eggs.

In *The Gift of Good Land,* Wendell Berry acknowledges the truth that *all* eating—even that of plant-based foods—involves a kind of death, a damage to the earth:

> To live, we must daily break the body and shed the blood of Creation. When we do this knowingly, lovingly, skillfully, reverently, it is a sacrament. When we do it ignorantly, greedily, clumsily, destructively, it is a *desecration.*[49]

It is possible to eat in ways that shed creation's blood and break its body reverently. It might mean spending a little more money to buy vegetables, eggs or meat from a local farmer or gardener, or it might mean spending more of your time with your hands in the dirt, coaxing your own food from the earth. Eating with joy while loving God's creation means humbly recognizing our place as members of creation, with a responsibility to cherish and protect biodiversity—in plants and animals. It means respecting animals as the divinely created subjects of their own lives while recognizing their legitimate use. It means remembering Eden and anticipating the new creation while living here and now. It can mean eating local, gardening, composting, recycling and more—but this will look different for city-dwellers as compared to country folk, as well as for the wealthier among us compared with those living on limited material resources.

At its heart, it means sitting down to the table mindful of God, respectful of the creation he loves, and believing that in eating this way—even if we're forgoing things we'd normally have—we are pursuing our own best good, our own greater joy.

One of the simplest ways to eat more sustainably is simply to waste less food. If you waste a loaf of bread, you waste not just the bread itself but all the resources that it took to bring that bread to you: the fuel for shipping the bread to the store, for producing the packaging, for heating the ovens, running the mixers, not to mention milling, harvesting and planting the grain. Looked at from this perspective, it is easy to understand why some people are passionate about food "rescue" on a large scale (check out foodrescue.org). Some people, known as "freegans," actively seek out and eat or redistribute edible food that has been discarded. On a more ordinary scale, many of our grandmothers and great-grandmothers, accustomed to hard times, passionately refused to waste food, repurposing leftovers into other dishes with mixed culinary success. Given that nearly as much edible food is thrown out as is eaten in the United States, one of the best things you can do to eat more sustainably is simply to waste less. Buy smaller packages, buy less at one time, check the cupboards before you go shopping or call for takeout. "Gather up the fragments," Jesus said, " . . . so that nothing may be lost" (Jn 6:12).

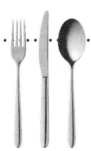

PRAYERS BEFORE EATING

O Lord, who clothes the lilies
And feeds the birds of the sky,
Who leads the lambs to pasture
And deer to the waterside,
Who multiplied loaves and fishes
And turned water into wine,
O Lord, join our table,
As guest and giver, to dine.
Amen.

Behind the loaf is the snowy flour;
Behind the flour is the mill;
Behind the mill is the sun and shower,
And the wheat and the Father's will.
Amen.

Praised are You, O God,
Guide of the Universe
Who creates innumerable living beings
And their needs, for all the things you have created to sustain them.
Praised are you, the life of the Universe.
Amen.
A Jewish prayer, from Saying Grace

We are happy
Because you have accepted us, dear Lord.
Sometimes we do not know what to do
With all our happiness.
We swim in your grace
Like a whale in the ocean.
The saying goes:
"An ocean never dries up,"
But we know your grace also never fails.
This food you have given us
Is one more proof.
Dear Lord,
Your grace is our happiness.
Hallelujah!
From Table Prayers—*a prayer from Africa*

Without Thy sunshine and Thy rain
We could not have the golden grain;
Without Thy love we'd not be fed;
We thank Thee for our daily bread.
Amen.

We thank you, Lord, for happy hearts
For rain and sunny weather
We thank you, Lord, for this our food
And that we are together.

. . . .

RECIPES

Sweet Potato (& Corn) Fritters
This is one of my family's new favorites, a new twist on our old
favorite, potato pancakes. Well, okay, my five-year-old isn't crazy
about them (yet). But the rest of us are. Fresh cilantro is expensive
(and likely imported) in the supermarket in wintertime, but it's
fairly easy to grow your own indoors. But don't leave it—or the
green onions—out. The orange, yellow and green in these make
them so pretty. If you're inclined to be snobbish about frozen
veggies, consider that few vitamins are lost during freezing, and
that commercially frozen foods are frozen at the peak of freshness.
You (and the planet) are way better off buying frozen veggies in
winter than buying fresh ones that have been shipped long distances. Plus, recently I've seen organic frozen corn everywhere
from Costco to Trader Joe's. If you planned ahead and froze corn
yourself in the summer, so much the better.

Grate **3 large sweet potatoes** (I don't bother to peel them if
they're organic, just scrub and grate). Mix with **1 cup frozen
corn kernels, rinsed, 4 chopped green onions, 4 tablespoons
chopped cilantro, 3 lightly beaten eggs and 1/3 cup whole
wheat flour.** (For non-gluten eaters substitute 2 tablespoons
cornstarch and 2 tablespoons potato flour.) Stir in about **1/2
teaspoon salt** and some **freshly ground black pepper.** Drop by
1/4 cupfuls into a pan well oiled with 1 part oil (preferably corn
or grapeseed) and 1 part butter—enough to keep them sizzling
but not floating. Cook about 3 minutes on each side, and keep
warm on a cookie sheet in a 275° oven while you cook the rest.

Serve with a simple sauce of juice from 3 limes, 1/2 teaspoon minced garlic, 1 teaspoon chopped cilantro, 1 tablespoon fish sauce (optional), 1 tablespoon soy sauce and 2 teaspoons sesame oil. Add chili flakes if you like things spicy, and please look for soy sauce that is just soy, wheat, salt and water; gluten-free eaters, look for tamari.[50]

Beef & Beer Stew

I began making this stew when we lived in Scotland, where the farmer's market and our local butcher carried beef from cattle raised on pasture. We were lucky enough to meet some of those local cattle whenever we hiked along the Fife Coastal path, where they grazed along rocky and hilly ground, patiently renewing the soil, converting grass into food for humans and delighting our children with their peaceful friendliness. Here in the US, we buy our meat from local farmers with the help of Localharvest.org.

Don't leave out the wine or the beer. It adds such a deep richness to the gravy. We like it best with the called-for Guinness, but I've also made it with gluten-free beer, so that it's safe for my gluten-free dad, and it's still fabulous.

Heat a large pot until a drop of water sizzles. Add 1/4 cup olive oil and 1 pound beef, cut into 1-inch pieces. Stir until brown and add 6 cloves of minced garlic. Cook 1 minute more and add 6 cups of beef stock or broth, 1 cup of Guinness beer, 1 cup red wine, 1 6-ounce can of tomato paste, 1 tablespoon each of sugar and dried thyme, 2-4 tablespoons Worcestershire sauce (I like lots) and 2 bay leaves. Simmer, covered, for 1 hour.

Meanwhile, in a separate pot, melt 1/2 stick (1/4 cup) butter. Add 3 pounds peeled and cubed russet potatoes, 1 large yellow onion, chopped, and 2 cups chopped, peeled carrots. Cover and simmer for 1 hour.

After both pots have simmered 1 hour, combine them in a

single pot and simmer for 30-45 minutes, until the flavors are well blended. Season with **salt** and **pepper**, stir in **2 tablespoons chopped fresh parsley**, and remove from heat. It's so delicious with no-knead bread or plain steamed rice and a glass of red wine, and just the thing for a cozy company meal on a winter's evening.[51]

• •

POINTS FOR ACTION

- Learn where you food comes from. *The Omnivore's Dilemma* is a good primer.

- Grow *something*, even if it's just some herbs in pots on the windowsill. There's nothing like watching unlikely looking little seeds grow from seedlings into something that can be part of your dinner. If at all possible, plant a garden.

- With the help of LocalHarvest.org, figure out what things are a part of your local (or local-*ish*) "foodshed." Even if you can't manage to eat mostly local foods (and few people can), every little step helps. As Steven Hopp notes in *Animal, Vegetable, Miracle*, if every US citizen ate just one meal a week (any meal) composed of locally and organically grown foods, it would reduce our country's oil consumption by over 1.1 million *barrels* (barrels!) of oil every week.

- Consider observing "meatless Mondays" (www.meatlessmonday .com; you could also go with pre-Vatican-II-style meatless Fridays!) as a way of cutting back on the amount of meat you eat—for your health, for the health of the planet and as a way of showing mercy to God's creatures, the animals.

- Learn about sustainable development projects in places that frequently face famine. Heifer International, Bread for the World and World Vision are particularly helpful resources for learning and action.

- Don't waste food! Buy only what you need, store leftovers carefully and do as the restaurants do: FIFO (first in, first out). In other words, organize your fridge and pantry to use things before they go bad!

6

Creative Eating

FOOD PREPARATION

AS CULTURE MAKING

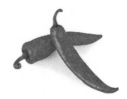

When my son Aidan was learning to talk, he called all breadlike things "bread"—tortillas were bread, toast was bread, focaccia was bread, *naan* and scones and muffins and baguettes were all bread to him, which makes sense. Each form of bread testifies to the similarities and differences between humans around the globe and how we've domesticated, cultivated and rendered various grains both edible and delicious.

Virtually everything we eat is as much a product of culture as of nature. We eat very few wild foods. Most of our food—whether from plant or animal—has been tamed. It's fashionable to idealize the "simpler" and more "natural" past, as do proponents of the Paleo diet, who insist that preagricultural foods were healthier. But despite this idealization of the primitive, a contemporary Paleo diet is made possible only by the workings of a globalized food system. Even the carrots and tomatoes you may grow in your own backyard are cultural products. In *Vegetables: A Biography*, Evelyne Bloch-Dano traces the history of vegetables like tomatoes, carrots and cabbages, showing how they have been "tamed" from their wild counterparts just as agricultural animals have—and how foods have embedded themselves into cultures in deeply significant ways. Where would Italian cuisine be without tomatoes, for example, or French food without potatoes?

Everywhere there are humans, there are different ways of doing things with food, and these distinctions have more than merely dietary significance. It's no accident that English people once referred derisively to the French as "frogs," while the French likewise called the English "roast beefs." Food is a mark of identity. "Tell me what you eat," goes the over-quoted line from Brillat-Savarin, "and I will tell you what you are."[1]

Food culture helps beget other cultural artifacts; the rise of agriculture marks the end of the hunter-gatherer existence as it marks the beginning of civilization-building—settled villages and towns, architecture, art and forms of economic exchange. Producing storable surpluses of food (like grain) makes possible the creation of settled civilizations. But no mere fuel to the production of "more important" culture and art, food itself is, and has always been, in virtually every place, deeply culturally significant. Ways of producing, preparing, sharing and serving food are important cultural and creative practices in their own right.

When my family shared a meal with our friends in Guatemala, for example, it would have been considered rude for the host of the dinner party not to offer his own plate to his guests, but it would have been equally rude of a guest to accept that offer. In *The Joy Luck Club*, Amy Tan tells the story of a deeply insulting comment made by a boyfriend eating a Chinese American mother's cooking.[2] "Not salty enough, no flavor!" the mother says, inviting the ritual protestations and assurances that the food she had cooked was good. "All it needs is a little soy sauce!" says the clueless American boyfriend. My grandmother felt that the "right" way to prepare chicken was to first rub it inside and out with salt, then rinse it with water before doing anything else. She was Jewish, and this was a way of koshering the meat, ensuring that no blood was left on it. But she didn't keep kosher; she was simply washing her chickens the way her mother had taught her, and her mother before her. And many people in the UK observe Pancake Day by eating pancakes with golden syrup on the Tuesday before Lent, whether or not they realize that the tradition was started hundreds of years ago in an effort to use up milk and eggs before the season of abstention from animal products.

Eating, like clothing and shelter, is a necessity, but just as every culture discovers and develops ways of building shelters and designing clothing that suits their particular needs and sensibilities, so too food and the exchanges that go with it stand as embodied articulations of our understanding of the world. "Foods," writes the neuro-anthropologist John S. Allen, "are cultural objects, invested implicitly and explicitly with meaning and significance beyond their nutritive value."[3]

Cooking is culture making, a way of making something of the world and an important cultural expression that all the prepared foods in the world can't replace. Food historian Harvey Levenstein notes that when commercial cake mixes first went on the market, they were unpopular because they required the baker to add only water. When the mixes were reengineered to require oil, eggs, and water or milk, consumers felt like there was more for them to do and liked the mixes much more.[4] We're created to be creative— to do things with our food to render it ever more edible and appealing—even if only in the simplified ways the industry prepares for us.

WHY PLEASURE MATTERS

I'd like to look at the fairly obvious notion that pleasure motivates culinary creativity, because I think that many Americans—and perhaps not least American Christians—have a long legacy of being suspicious of pleasure in eating, and this has shaped our approach to eating in not entirely salutary ways. We live in a culture that is on the one hand full of foods that are engineered for maximum pleasure and on the other full of nutritional advice that warns us of the dangers of such pleasure. One doctor who advocates a vegan diet cowrote the ominously titled book *The Pleasure Trap*. Early in the life of the church, Christian writers were anxious about the body's appetites. St. Gregory of Nyssa, one of the Cappodocian fathers (c. 335-c. 395), wrote on the five or six ways in which a person could be "gluttonous," a hairsplitting, angst-producing collection picked up later by the none-too-svelte Thomas Aquinas, including such sins as eating "too eagerly" or "too wildly." A wariness of pleasure has marked Christian attitudes toward food from the time of St. Gregory and St. Augustine to today. A recent bestseller, *Made to Crave,* follows in this line, seeing all cravings for food as essentially dangerous and potentially sinful because we are "made to crave" *God.* For Lysa TerKeurst, the ideal is to eat only the healthiest food possible— the pleasure of eating is in this view an intellectual pleasure of doing the "right thing" for one's body.[5]

Christian wariness of pleasure in food, while certainly not universal, has had particular importance in the United States. Relative to the United State's brief history as a nation, its history of dietary asceticism is long and intertwined with its religious history, and seems also to be deeply connected to faddish obsessions with perfecting health through dietary discipline. The first prominent American vegetarian was a clergyman named William Metcalfe, who established a church in Philadelphia in 1817, promoting the idea that it was the eating of animal flesh that brought about the fall.[6] Sylvester Graham (of graham cracker fame) was also a vegetarian, a temperance advocate and a Presbyterian minister who advocated an abstemious diet based on homemade brown bread. He believed fervently that the consumption of flesh led to all kinds of sins, especially sexual sins. This belief was echoed by Dr. John Harvey Kellogg, founder of the Battle Creek Sanitarium, a diet-, exercise- and enema-centered getaway in Michigan.

When I was in college and editing a small student journal, a nutrition student submitted an essay arguing that eating for health was much more important than eating for pleasure, bolstering her argument with Bible verses. Without knowing precisely why, I was repelled by the piece, perhaps because it made explicit a doctrine I lived by but still hated.

Once, when I still feared pleasure in food as potentially dangerous, I tried to make macaroni and cheese. But instead of good old-fashioned elbow pasta, I used whole wheat noodles. Instead of whole milk, I used soy milk. I did put a bit of real cheese in there but cut the amount by three-quarters and replaced the rest with pureed carrot. It was awful, truly awful, and not the kind of accidental awful that happens to every cook occasionally. It was awful by design, awful because it wasn't intended to bring enjoyment— it was intended to be *healthy*.

Maybe it was, in a limited sense, nourishing—bringing necessary vitamins, minerals and energy to the body and staving off hunger pangs. Certainly I was grateful to have it. It was a better meal than many people in the world would enjoy that night. But it certainly wasn't satisfying in itself. If it was satisfying at all, it was only because of an *idea*: "I'm doing something that's good for my body by ingesting this." This kind of cooking—cooking that is motivated by an idea, rather than by the wondrous materials of food— is a kind of asceticism, an exaltation of a idea (in this case, healthfulness) over pleasure, and indeed, over the sensory experience of food and eating. This approach to food is, as Robert Farrar Capon wrote, an "intellectual fad, imposing a handful of irrelevant philosophical prejudices on a grandly material business."

Eating *is* grandly material business—one of the important ways in which the body interfaces with the outside world, which is why it has been the site of so much conflict and angst for people of faith throughout the ages. But does the same God who calls us to his kingdom with words like "Listen carefully to me, and eat what is good, and delight yourselves in rich food" (Is 55:2) also call us to dietary asceticism, to perfect adherence to regimens of health?

One reason I object to the notion that God is most pleased by "healthy eating" is because what constitutes healthy eating is not agreed on in all times or in all places and, indeed, is a new concept. Nutrition, as any good nutritionist will tell you, is a young science, its research and principles having begun a mere hundred years or so ago.[7] But that hasn't stopped nutritionists, doctors and others from churning out books outlining the "right" diet, sometimes even using the Bible to argue for their positions, whether raw veganism in *The Hallelujah Diet*, organic omnivory in *The Maker's Diet* or periodic "cleansing" fasts in *What Would Jesus Eat?* Even where Christian diet books reject secular motivations for weight-loss (like looking good), they do not challenge the powerful discourses of health that insist eating is primarily about maintaining optimal bodily health.

Certainly, what we eat matters to our health and functioning; Morgan Spurlock's experiment in *Super Size Me* showed that pretty clearly. But a preoccupation with the "rightness" or "wrongness" of foods can also lead to an illness of soul that prevents us from receiving food as a pleasurable gift. I think our *experience* of food can—and perhaps should—be one of *enjoyment* and *encounter*. Of course there are ways of eating that do very little good to anyone; without question, there are foods that, consumed inordinately, cause harm. My beloved great-uncle *loved* food, all food, and ate plenty of it, even after he was diagnosed with diabetes. When he died of a heart attack in his late fifties, his wife was devastated and even a little angry: "Why couldn't he change his diet? We might still have him with us if he had." We need an understanding of pleasure that is tempered by moderation but that still celebrates *pleasure* in the grandly material business of eating.

THE PLEASURE OF PAYING ATTENTION

The Episcopal priest Robert Farrar Capon wrote a witty, wise and prescient book about cooking in the 1960s titled *The Supper of the Lamb*. An oft-cited early chapter instructs the reader to enjoy a long encounter with an onion. That's right: an onion. He recommends setting aside an hour, at least, for peeling, chopping, observing and finally cooking the onion. It's a strange chapter, to be sure, but once you've really explored the onion, gotten to know the onion for what it is, it is difficult to look at an onion dismissively again. The point of this bizarre little exercise is repeated throughout the book—that we too seldom encounter things as things *in themselves*. We look at them for what they *mean*, or for what they mean *to us*. So a cherry is not a shiny orb of tangy sweetness grown from a beautiful tree blossom, but a five-calorie delivery system for antioxidants, vitamin C, potassium, iron, fiber and magnesium. This, Capon says, is idolatry, a concept he returns to again and again:

> Every time [a person] diagrams something instead of looking at it, every time he regards not what a thing is but what it can be made to mean to him, reality slips away from him and he is left with nothing but the oldest monstrosity in the world— an idol.[8]

One of Capon's favorite idols to destroy is the calorie. Calories are nothing at all, he says, just "invisible little spooks." And if you think about it, it's true. You've never eaten a calorie in your life. Neither have I nor anyone else, because a calorie is nothing more than a unit of heat energy. *One calorie equals the amount of heat energy that it takes to heat one gram of water one degree Celsius.* That's it.

Even so, calories—units of measure logically equivalent to, say, horsepower—became, not long after they were discovered, a dirty word, something to fear and avoid. The Weight Watchers program (always some variation on the theme of a very low-calorie diet) instructs its participants to scrupulously measure various numerical values of what they consume. Capon's point is that all these are abstractions. They are not real things. They force you to take the real thing (food) and measure it, compute it, portion it and track it irrespective of any of its essential, created qualities. Calories and abstracted diets are nothing but diagrams; and "one real thing," Capon insists, "is closer to God than all the diagrams in the world."[9]

Cooking and eating with joyful attentiveness can elevate food from mere fuel—which it never really is, anyway—to a celebration of creation and what it means to be human.

Despite all that dietary asceticism in its various forms may preach, taste buds and the distinct categories of taste (salty, sweet, sour, bitter and *umami*, or savory), to say nothing of the wonders of texture and temperature, convince me that eating is about so much more than survival. To paraphrase Remy, the rat-who-would-be-chef in the animated film *Ratatouille*:"Humans don't just survive—they *live!*" While all his relatives were content to fill their bellies with any old thing they could scavenge from other people's garbage, Remy loved to smell, taste, combine and create with food. More than fuel for survival, food to him was a life-affirming experience and an act of passionate creativity. The film does a masterful job of showing how Remy experiences food as aesthetically thrilling in ways barely comprehensible to his rat relatives. When Remy tastes a strawberry and some cheese, he sees brilliant colors and hears soaring melodies; when he tastes them in combination, he sees fireworks and hears a symphony. By contrast, his brother, tasting the same stuff, experiences only a short burst of color and hears a few weak notes. Thus fine ingre-

dients were to the rat-chef like oil paints in the hands of a master
painter, musical tones in the hands of a composer.

When I interviewed two of New York's finest chefs, Claudia
Fleming and Gerry Hayden of the North Fork Table and Inn, I
discovered that the fictional depiction of Remy was very true to
the dedication, artistry and enthusiasm of these fine chefs. Although many chefs do not self-identify as artists, preferring to
think of themselves as hard-working people who have mastered a
craft, I have little doubt that they are artists in every sense. For
one thing, they'd rather go broke than offer their guests anything
less than the absolute best quality ingredients prepared in the
finest, freshest way. As Dorothy Sayers wrote, they "live dangerously" out of respect for their work. I was also surprised and delighted at the joy that the chefs take in particulars—in the raw
materials, the foods!—that call forth their artistry. Both left lu-
crative positions in New York City restaurants to come to the East
End of Long Island, where vineyards and small biodynamic farms
line the country roads, because here, says Chef Hayden, you find
"peaches that *really* taste like peaches." He shaped his hands
around an imaginary peach and closed his eyes. "*This,* this in-
spires me to create," he said.[10]

Yet even everyday cooking can reflect God's own creative work
when we pay attention to every bit of food that comes before us
with loving attention, regarding it for what it *is* in all its quirky
uniqueness. As the Reverend Capon insisted, our real work "is to
look at the things of the world and to love them for *what they are.*
That is, after all, what God does and man was not made in God's
image for nothing."[11] A peach is a peach with its own texture, taste
and smell—not a number of calories or a set of antioxidants. Or,
to use a non-food example, a game of basketball is not a set of statistics noting rebounds, points and turnovers; a desire to see a
good basketball game isn't satisfied by hearing the stats. By giving
loving consideration to our food, eating can become an act of

worship as we regard what God has made and appreciate it for what it is, both in its independence from us and for the delightful use that we can make of it.

In order to appreciate the wonderful creativity present even in the simplest cooking, we must try to look at food and cooking as if for the first time, not seeing a recipe or a dish as natural and inevitable but as the product of ingenuity and creativity and the miracle of soil fertility and divine blessing. Even basic cooking involves a kind of creative alchemy, an altering of substances by the application of heat and other physical processes like grinding and chopping, and chemical processes like soaking and combining. Think of the endless possibilities that start with just a handful of basic ingredients: how many different kinds of bread there are, how many ways to prepare rice or noodles. The world over, people have ancient and time-honored customs regarding food, which are inextricably linked to their culture, their way of using their God-given creativity to shape the world around them. The ways in which we take raw materials—salt, milk, tomatoes, olives, basil—and turn them into something delicious, beautiful and life-sustaining (a tomato-mozzarella-basil salad with olive oil, for example) is ordinary, and yet extraordinary.

Surely we don't *have* to cook to enjoy eating, do we? In the strictest sense, no. But I *do* think that knowing more about the food you eat, how it's raised and prepared makes eating it a fuller and more pleasurable experience. Such awareness and attention is, to my mind, Godlike. God as Creator delights to look on the creation with deep understanding, knowledge and love. To the degree that we cook from scratch and understand the ingredients we're working with and the dynamics of their interaction with each other and with heat, we celebrate the riches of God's creation and exercise our divinely crafted faculties for beauty and creativity. Never mind that most of us will always be amateurs in the kitchen. "Amateur," which comes from the Old French meaning for "lover of," is just what we're meant to be, as Capon writes, "[The amateur] look[s] the world back to grace."[12] We live the new creation, in other words, by cherishing the creation—all of it—and using our faculties for culture-making. As Dorothy Sayers wrote, "A work of creation is a work of love."[13]

The culture in which most of us live allows us to cook very little or not at all. A few years ago, the U.S. Department of Agriculture's Economic Research Service estimated that Americans spend nearly half of their food dollars away from home—a higher percentage than any on record. These numbers reflect many things, among them more and more people working more and more hours away from home, inexpensive and easily accessible restaurant foods, and a general decline in the value placed on a "home cooked meal." America has been moving away from from-scratch cooking for a long time; in the post–World War II years, the development of processed, prepared and packaged foods changed the way Americans cooked. By now most of us have heard *too many times* that processed food is "bad" for our bodies, but that's not what I primarily have in view here.

As strange as this may sound, I do believe that there is a countercultural and deeply redemptive aspect to gardening and cooking from scratch. This isn't to say that I believe it's wrong to order in pizza or pop open a can now and then—of course not! However, I do think that overemphasizing speed and convenience can rob us of the sense that food is important—a way in which God extends loving care to us—and an important way for us to practice God-given creativity while celebrating God's own creation.[14]

One year, I decided to make the classic mushroom-soup green-bean casserole, but instead of buying cans of soup, fried onions and green beans, I decided to create it from fresh ingredients. What were the essential flavors and textures I wanted to preserve or improve upon? I wanted to use fresh green beans, and to have a more natural creamy taste that came from real cream, not "canned cream-of-something." I wanted real onions, not processed ones, and so on. I rediscovered the basic white sauce, which is what canned cream soups mimic. I added fresh mushrooms and played with the technique and ingredients until I'd come up with a dish that did the important work of calling forth the memory of the processed food "classic" while standing on its own merits. Now I make it every year for Thanksgiving.

It wasn't until the Industrial Revolution that work was, for so many people, moved out of the sphere of home and field. Before then, the business of living and making a living depended heavily on diverse kinds of creative production, much of it centered on food. Sure, lots of drudgery was involved in the homesteading life (just read about butter churning in *Little House in the Big Woods*!), but there was tremendous creative satisfaction as well—and I refer you to that same book again if you doubt it! While I'm grateful for the opportunities allowed by a specialized economy—like the chance to write this book because I *don't* have to spend all my time feeding and clothing myself and my family—I'm not alone in my hunch that one's quality of life is diminished if one doesn't have the opportunity to exercise a relatively broad range of skills in the course of living.[15] Furthermore, *not* producing generally means you're consuming instead. And while being a consumer is a necessary part of living in an economy like ours, it's not, ultimately, what we're created to be. We're astonishing creatures, capable of creativity that ranges from the ordinary wonder of a perfectly flaky pie crust to the extraordinary brilliance of a Bernini sculpture.

Not creating has another significant effect on us. When we're used to being on the consumer end of something rather than having at least practiced producing for ourselves, it's harder for us to understand what has or has not gone into its production. I'll give you a silly example.

Some years ago I became a knitting fanatic, rapidly learning in a short time how to knit, purl, create ribs, cables, lace and how to craft seamless garments by knitting "in the round." Once I became familiar with the various methods for producing knitwear, I was unable to look at sweaters, hats, mittens and other knitted items in the same way. I would look at a simple sweater in a shop and say to myself, "Hm, so they cast on with a garter stitch for two inches, changing to stockinette punctuated by K2togs/YOs every other row every fifth stitch." That reads like utter nonsense to non-knitters, but it serves as an example for how producing and creating something changes your perspective on the thing that's for most people an object of consumption. Which is another way of saying it's hard for us to judge quality cooking if we ourselves are not somewhat familiar with cooking.

I have an unscientific hunch that people who love to cook love to eat and tend to eat with greater enthusiasm and relish than those who don't cook. Why? Because our taste buds are trained to recognize certain flavors and textures, and because we take an interest in the experience of eating related to the techniques involved in creating the sensations we're experiencing. Paying close attention to the processes involved in preparing food makes it possible for us to enjoy our food more than we would otherwise. And paying close attention to food—in the preparation and in the eating—heightens our enjoyment by teaching us where the idols lie.

As I've mentioned, nutritional concerns can be idols, as in "Eat your salmon, it's got lots of Omega-3s," or "I hate this cereal but it's got a lot of fiber" or "This croissant from the French bakery is the best I've ever tasted, but it's going to make me fat." In each of these remarks, the eater reveals that it's not the food itself that she's encountering or inviting the other to encounter, but an idea, in this case, *healthfulness*. Associations with food (which are frequently exploited in advertisements) are also potential idols. When you're sick or anxious, don't you tend to want the "comfort foods" of your childhood, not so much for their taste but for the warm feelings they create by triggering certain memories? A holiday Cheerios commercial showing Grandma demonstrating the distance between her house and her grandchild's house with cereal pieces subconsciously trains you to associate the supposedly unassuming Cheerio with warm Grandma feelings—you reach for them with thoughts and feelings of what they *represent* more than what they *are.*

Next time you have a sudden food craving, examine it for the possible associations (whether ad-connected or not) and ask yourself if it's the food or the *idea* of the food that you're really craving. (My irrational craving is packaged ramen noodles. Every so often I think I want them so badly, and then when I taste them, I don't like them. It's the idea, the association, the fun that my friend and I used to have preparing and eating them when we were all of eight years old.)[16] Big money is made from happy associations. Just think of the myriad ways in which McDonald's Corporation has worked to make the experience of eating McDonald's a "happy experience"—Ronald McDonald, Playplaces and, of course, the Happy Meal, to say nothing of the hundreds of commercials promising warm human connection by way of the Golden Arches. ("You deserve a break today.") If we stop to think about what McDonald's is selling—cheap, highly processed food—we know it's unhealthy for us and destructive to the planet. But the kind of pleasure it offers is the kind that depends on ignorance, not understanding. It is focused on consumption, while pleasurable, it *isn't* joyful eating.

So I believe that to eat with joy, we must eat creatively, and to do that, it's a good idea to learn how to cook from scratch, encountering the wonders of God's creation and human agriculture while creating your own bit of kitchen culture. Cooking can keep you healthier and happier, especially when you cook and eat with others, making real human connections, not the counterfeit marketing-associated pseudo-connections! (Barbara Kingsolver notes that she's given and received some of "life's most important hugs" in the kitchen, and many people find that their own memories are full of warm associations with food and kitchens.) Cooking also helps keep us from eating at the end of the food industry pipeline. While it's all but impossible to ascertain the natural history of a meal at Applebee's (except to say that a fair portion of what's on your plate has come from or through an industrial park), it's more than possible to cook meals for yourself from ingredients whose provenance you know with some degree of certainty and even intimacy.

Additionally, as you learn the practical art of cooking alchemy, gaining greater understanding of the subtle actions and interactions of one ingredient with another, you will also refine your God-given sense of taste and be able to fine-tune your recipes and techniques to best suit your sensibilities. (And that's really fun, not to mention tasty.)

Maybe you're thinking, *But I'm not a good cook,* or *But I hate cooking,* or *I don't have the time to cook* or simply, *I don't know where to begin!* While I can't anticipate and answer all of your anxieties about cooking, a few words are in order. First, I do believe that *anyone* can learn to cook reasonably well, and that doing it more and more frequently can help it become an enjoyable activity. To the question of time, I'd point out that few things are as sustaining in every sense as learning to feed yourself well and that a decent home-cooked meal doesn't have to take too long to prepare. The more you cook, the easier and faster it's likely to become. And, finally, as to the question of not knowing where to begin, I'd say this: start by watching a good cook, ideally, a cook that you know in real life, but even TV chefs (check out the old episodes of Julia Child on *The French Chef*) can be good teachers. And, of course, you can start with a good cookbook of a cuisine or style that you know you like.

One challenge my family and I have undertaken is to eat locally and in season as much as possible. To that end, we shop at farm stands and farmer's markets and grow a good amount of vegetables (and potatoes) in our own backyard. Our eggs come from a woman who keeps hens in her backyard and reuses the same egg cartons dozens of times. We order roasts and other cuts of meat from a local farmer who keeps her animals on pasture. I'm one of those insane people who cans jams and pickles and peaches in the brutal summer heat, and I intentionally grow *way* too many green beans so that there will be plenty to pack away in my freezer for the winter. Is eating this way a challenge? Well, kind of. It means a little more planning and a good bit of work, but the quality and flavor of our food more than makes up for it. I'm in agreement with the Slow Food movement's ethos, which is playful rather than dour: they're all about *enjoying* the best possible taste of food, which sometimes means waiting until spring to have a green salad. But there's a valuable lesson to be learned there. Barbara Kingsolver likens it to teaching young people about keeping their virginity:

> Only if they wait to experience intercourse under the ideal circumstances (the story goes), will they know its true value. *"Blah blah blah,"* hears the teenager: words issuing from a mouth that can't even wait . . . to satisfy a craving for everything *now*. We're raising our children on the definition of promiscuity if we feed them a casual, indiscriminate mingling of foods from every season plucked from the supermarket, ignoring how our sustenance is cheapened by wholesale desires.
>
> *Waiting for the quality experience* seems to be the constitutional article that has slipped from American food custom.[17]

Kingsolver and her family made a yearlong experiment of eating only locally produced food, and though they went into it with some trepidation—thinking of all the things that they were not going to be able to have—they finished the year and decided to keep eating local, so great was their enjoyment of their new way of living: "When we changed our thinking [away from dwelling on what they *couldn't* have] and started every meal with the question, 'What *do* we have? What's in season? What do we have plenty of?'—it became a long exercise in gratitude."[18]

Setting a limit on your food consumption (e.g., we're going to eat X number of meals a week from local ingredients only) can be a catalyst for creativity and greater enjoyment. Creativity actually flourishes given a degree of limitation. (You may, wrote G. K. Chesterton, "free a tiger from his bars, but do not free him from his stripes."[19]) It's no accident that tomatoes, basil and olive oil go well together and strike most of us as essentially Italian, or that traditional New England dishes include slow-baked beans with maple syrup and seafood chowders with potatoes—those specific places, their cultures and their climates make those kinds of meals possible, and the same is true of Californian, Canadian and Cajun cuisines. Your region may or may not have a distinctive cooking style arising from its own particular culture, climate and sensibility. In any case, the best place to begin may be at the farmer's market or in your garden, encountering those onions or potatoes or beans or *whatever*.

An additional unexpected benefit of eating seasonally and gardening is that it has given us much greater awareness of the turning of the seasons and of the weather. While it would be a stretch to say that this practice returns us to the agricultural mindset shared by people in the ancient Near East (the background of the Bible), it wouldn't be that far off either. In our world of twenty-four-hour supermarkets with abundances of *everything now*—grapes from Chile, lettuce from Mexico, kiwis from New Zealand, beef from Argentina, oranges from Costa Rica—intentionally returning to a way of eating that follows the seasons and the weather grounds us more completely in the place where we live, links us more significantly to the God-ordained rhythms of rain and sunshine, cold and heat, humidity and drought.

When strawberries were (finally!) in season, my husband and I took our berry-loving boys to a local u-pick operation and let them pick to their hearts' content. "Is it really strawberry time? Wow!" said my five-year-old son, who by now is used to me explaining why we won't buy imported berries in January, and who has learned to wait until the right season for strawberries.

(Once, he fell down half a flight of stairs, and, though he seemed fine, he was rubbing his leg, and in my typical anxious-mom way I kept asking, "Are you okay? Does it hurt?" Finally, exasperated, he said, "Mom! It feels like strawberries-not-in-season taste! They taste like nothing! It feels. Like. Nothing!" Point taken.)

When it's strawberry time, we let them go crazy, eating strawberries at every meal if that's what they want. This summer, as we bent among the rows of strawberry plants together, gathering the ripe, delicious berries, snacking on them now and then, we were fully present in that time, in that place, filled with wonder and delight at the God who turns the seasons and the day and night with glorious regularity. At the same time we saved plenty to make our own strawberry jam—which gives the bread eaten in winter a delicious bit of spreadable summer, a wonderful way to remember the beauty and bounty of God's earth even when it's covered with gray clouds and piles of snow.

Starting with ingredients—the fresh and delicious food that's available around you—is very different than starting with recipes and requires more from the cook than slavish obedience to those recipes. That's why I (and many far better cooks than I) recommend familiarizing yourself with the basics of cooking techniques. None other than Julia Child wrote that "once you have mastered a technique, you barely have to look at a recipe again."[20] Technique—knowing how (and why and when) to marinate, dredge, sauté, broil, roast, braise, steam, cream or bake some-thing—lets you take what you have (zucchini, perhaps) and make something delicious out of it (zucchini fritters), even if you don't have or can't find a recipe.

Mastering technique, of course, is almost impossible without first following someone else's recipe. The books I've found most helpful in this way include Julia Child's *Mastering the Art of French Cooking* and all the books from America's Test Kitchen, including *The New Best Recipe*, *The Best International Recipe* and a number of others. These books offer detailed explanations on *why* each recipe is formulated and executed as it is. The *Best Recipe* books offer many mini science lessons that teach you how given ingredients act and interact with each other to produce a certain kind of taste and texture. In a similar but less practical vein, Harold McGee's classic book *On Food and Cooking: The Science and Lore of the Kitchen* offers fascinatingly detailed expla-nations of seemingly ordinary kitchen happenings—what's hap-pening biochemically when you scramble an egg, melt butter or beat pancake batter, and how it affects what the end result tastes, smells and feels like.

While some of this is more than you need to know to be a good home cook, I've found that knowing the *why* has greatly improved my cooking and allowed me to improvise based on what I've got on hand at a given moment. It has certainly helped me to appre-ciate good cooking even more and to figure how to improve recipes I already know and love. Moreover, even though I was not espe-cially stellar at science at school, I'm deeply fascinated by the hands-on biology and chemistry of the kitchen—gardening, choosing produce and cooking have become for me another way of delighting deeply in God as I exercise the faculties of creativity that God has entrusted to me. As Capon wrote:

Never stop cultivating the virtue of paying attention to the uniqueness of every last morsel that comes before you. The world we live in exists not because it is an old inventory item once made and long since shelved, but because each scrap of its marvelous being is an intimate and immediate response to the Creator who, at every moment, romances it out of nothing into existence by loving regard.[21]

Cooking in a way that delights the senses may *seem* less important than practicing eating together, choosing foods produced in ways that are respectful of people and God's planet, and giving thanks to the Creator. But cooking—and learning to cook well—enhances each of these things. A single delicious meal transformed Julia Child from bored housewife to, well, Julia Child—and she remembered that meal all her life with a sense of wonder and excitement. She and others have written eloquently and extensively on the pleasures of scrumptious food eaten with friends. Great meals are social glue and create bonds between people.

Cooking your own food also allows you to know with greater certainty that what you're eating has been produced in a way that's respectful to other people and to God's creation. It exercises your senses and faculties in praise of the Creator who has given you those gifts of sense and ability as well as the tasty and fragrant materials—foods!—on which to exercise them creatively for your delight and that of those around you. No unnecessary garnish to human fuel-ups, taste, as Capon wrote, points us toward God's lavish goodness and grace, cooking and eating readying us for the Supper of the Lamb:

> Man invented cooking before he thought of nutrition. To be sure, food keeps us alive, but that is only its smallest and most temporary work. Its eternal purpose is to furnish our sensibilities against the day when we shall sit down at the heavenly banquet and see how gracious the Lord is. . . .

Nourishment is only necessary for a while; what we shall need forever is taste. . . . Food is the daily sacrament of unnecessary goodness, ordained for a continual remembrance that the world will always be more delicious than it is useful. Necessity is the mother only of clichés. It takes playfulness to make poetry.[22]

PRAYERS BEFORE MEALS

Lord, you are faithful in all your words
and kind in all your works.
You uphold all who are falling and
raise up all who are bowed down.
With our eyes we look to you, O Lord,
You give us our food in due season.
The eyes of all look to you,
and you give them their food in due season.
You open your hand;
you satisfy the desire of every living thing.
You are righteous in your ways
and kind in all your works.
Help us to bless your name this day and forever.
Amen.
Based on Psalm 145

Great God, the Giver of all good,
Accept our praise and bless our food.
Grace, health, and strength to us afford
Through Jesus Christ, our blessed Lord.
Amen.

O Lord Jesus Christ, without whom nothing is sweet or savory, we ask you to bless our food, and with your blessed presence, to cheer our hearts, that in all our eating and drinking we may taste your

goodness to your honor and glory. Amen.
Adapted from King Henry VIII's English Primer

. . . .
RECIPES

Cinnamon Rolls

Cinnamon rolls are one of those foods that have been so re-created by the food industry so as to bear but a shadowy resemblance to the real thing. These rolls are treats, to be sure, but they are *real* food. Enjoy them with coffee and friends.

Dissolve **1 heaping tablespoon of dry yeast** in **1/4 cup of warm—not hot—water**. Set aside.

Melt **1 stick (1/2 cup) butter**, and stir in **1/3 cup sugar** (I like to use organic fair-trade evaporated cane juice). Stir in **1 cup of whole milk** that's been warmed slightly, **1 beaten egg**, **2 teaspoons pure vanilla extract** and **1 1/2 teaspoon salt**. To this add the yeast-water mixture. Gradually stir in **4 to 5 cups bread flour** (up to half whole-wheat), changing the stirring to kneading once necessary. Knead 5-10 minutes, or until the dough is smooth and elastic. Wipe dough all over with butter, cover and set aside for 1 hour.

Meanwhile, mix together **1/2 cup firmly packed brown sugar** and **2 to 2 1/2 tablespoons ground cinnamon**. Set aside. Soften **another stick (1/2 cup) butter** and set aside.

When the dough has risen, gently push it down and begin to stretch and pull it to fit an 11" x 15" baking sheet. Take your time and push it down evenly. Using a pastry brush (or your clean fingers), spread softened butter all over the dough, except for the long side that is farthest from you, leaving a 1" x 15" strip CLEAN. Then carefully spread the cinnamon sugar over the butter. Roll up from bottom edge *loosely*—not firmly—and use the "clean" edge to seal up the roll. Saw the log very gently with a serrated knife into 1 1/2-inch pieces. (It helps to score the log lightly before you cut.) Lay the slices almost touching in a buttered 9" x 13" pan. Cover and allow the rolls to rise for an hour. While you wait, make the frosting by creaming together **2 ounces cream cheese, 1/4 cup of butter, 1 cup of powdered sugar** and **1 teaspoon pure vanilla extract.** When the rolls have risen again, bake at 350° for 15-20 minutes. Tip onto a large plate immediately, and when slightly cooled, spread with frosting. Yum.

Potato Pancakes

The Hanukkah favorite, perfect throughout the winter! My kids and husband like them with ketchup—they're kind of like a hash brown then, but I (and my parents) love them with the more Eastern European toppings of sour cream and applesauce. Either way, they're cheap, filling and really tasty.

Grate (if they're organic, just leave the skins on) **3 large potatoes** and squeeze in a clean cloth to release some of their liquid. Mix with **1/4 cup flour, 2 eggs** and **1 large yellow onion, finely chopped.** If it looks soupy, add a bit more flour. Add about **1 teaspoon salt** and some **fresh black pepper.** Drop by 1/4 cupfuls into a hot pan oiled with 1 part oil (preferably corn or grapeseed) and 1 part butter—enough to keep them sizzling but not floating. Drain on paper towels, if necessary, and keep warm in a 275° oven. Serve immediately.

Ratatouille-like-the-Movie

Chef Thomas Keller created this dish when he consulted with Pixar Studios on the film *Ratatouille*. I shamelessly capitalized on the appeal of the rat-chef Remy to get my five-year-old to eat lots of vegetables by cooking ratatouille in a simplified version of Keller's recipe so that it would look like the dish in the film. (I'm not recommending the film for young viewers. My young boy knew about Remy from a library book he found that was a movie tie-in. The film has some really scary sequences.)

1 1/2 peppers (red, yellow, orange or purple, seeded, ribbed and chopped finely)

1/2 cup finely chopped yellow onion

1 teaspoon minced garlic

1 sprig each of thyme and parsley (or a pinch each of the dried herbs)

1 bay leaf

Sauté in **2 tablespoons extra virgin olive oil** until the onions begin to caramelize; then add **3 finely chopped tomatoes.**

Cook down for 10 or 15 minutes, stirring frequently. Add salt to taste, then spread the sauce in the bottom of an ovenproof dish (about 9" x 13"), reserving 1 tablespoon of the sauce.

Slice into very thin rounds (you may want to try and select vegetables of similar diameter for visual appeal):

1 long zucchini

1 Japanese (skinny) eggplant

1 yellow squash similar in diameter and length to the zucchini

4 Roma tomatoes (or other dense, smallish tomatoes)

Arrange the vegetables in the pan on top of the sauce, alternating 1 slice of zucchini, 1 slice eggplant, 1 slice yellow squash, 1 slice tomato—repeat, going back and forth or around and around in the dish, overlapping the vegetables so that each just peeks out behind the other.

Bake, covered with a lid or with foil, in a preheated 275° degree oven for 2 hours, then uncover and bake 30 minutes more. There should not be much liquid in the pan after the last 30 minutes of baking; if there is, put it on the stove on low heat to reduce the liquid. (This long, slow baking develops the flavor of the vegetables and gives them a great texture.)

Meanwhile, combine the tablespoon of reserved sauce with:

1 tablespoon extra virgin olive oil

1 teaspoon balsamic vinegar

Some fresh herbs (like chervil, thyme, basil or parsley)

Season with **salt** and **pepper** to taste, and use as a vinaigrette to drizzle over the warm ratatouille. Couscous or quinoa cooked in broth is a delicious side dish with this unusual but tasty dish.

• •

POINTS FOR ACTION

• Spring might be the best season to begin searching around for local foods: asparagus, broccoli, lettuces and strawberries are all at their freshest and most delicious.

• Try one new from-scratch recipe a week.

• Cook with friends! Chances are you know someone who is an avid cook—or perhaps even a chef. Plan an afternoon and/or evening of cooking and eating together.

• Be playful in your cooking! What different kinds of salsas and chutneys could you create based on the fruits that are available where you live?

• Read about the science of cooking, and let the intricacies of God's creation present in even the homeliest of acts surprise you.

• Slow down. The pleasures of eating are as much in the mind as in the mouth. Try to experience your food with all your senses.

7

· ·

Redemptive Eating

PUTTING BEST PRACTICES TOGETHER

IN THE REAL WORLD

When people find out that I write about food and eating from a Christian perspective, their initial response is usually to apologize for their own dietary practices. Either that, or they assume that I'm a big fan of *The Maker's Diet, The Hallelujah Diet* or *What Would Jesus Eat?* I always feel awkward when the subject of my writing comes up in conversations taking place over meals—especially meals at other people's houses where I'm a guest. Almost without fail, people assume that I am about to pronounce judgment on their eating habits in general or on the meal they are about to serve me. People who don't know me well—or who've never watched me cook—seem to think that I survive entirely on homegrown vegetables and sunshine, when in fact there hasn't been an American who loved butter more since Julia Child passed away. At any given moment, my freezer holds upwards of 8 pounds of it! If I happen to let on about my passion for butter, I inevitably hear something like this: "But I thought butter was bad for you? Aren't animal fats unhealthy?"

Thanks to many different factors—not least, news media grasping for fodder for sensational stories ("Eat your veggies" doesn't make a compelling headline), food industry lobbyists keeping government agencies from saying anything against their products and nutrition studies funded by industry—we Americans are confused about what to eat. (Butter—an ancient agricultural product loaded with saturated fat?—or margarine—a feat of the laboratory that's cholesterol-free?)

One of the confounding factors in these discussions is what Marion Nestle calls "nutrient-by-nutrient" nutrition, which goes something like this: a study comes out indicating that the red wine consumed by the French seems to offer some protection against heart disease, possibly due to certain compounds known as resverotrols. Suddenly, American laboratories are scrambling to create red-wine supplement pills, Kashi is adding it to their cereals and consumers are buying the stuff, apparently believing that these supplements will offer the same (or similar) benefits to actually drinking red wine.

Nestle writes: "The problem with nutrient-by-nutrient science is that it *takes the nutrient out of the context of the food, the food out of the context of the diet, and the diet out of the context of the lifestyle.*"

It's probably impossible to isolate magic compounds and put them into supplemental pills and potions that do anyone any good. Numerous studies have indicated that vitamin and mineral supplementation doesn't work—and, in some cases, may even cause harm. Skim milk was (and is) considered by many to be more "healthful" than whole milk due to the same assumptions about milk fat that cause some to demonize butter—but some research suggests that the fat in milk may actually have important anti-cancer properties that men, especially, omit at their peril.

See how quickly things get confusing?

Nutrition is a young science; there are few things nutritionists can state with anything close to certainty. Eating whole, unprocessed foods—fruits, vegetables and whole grains—in something close to their "natural" states (i.e., not "fruit snacks," not "veggie chips") is fairly uncontroversial. But beyond that, as Michael Pollan argues persuasively in his book *In Defense of Food*, diets of astonishing variety—vegetarian, carnivorous, omnivorous and everything in between—can be very healthy. In any case, isolating this or that "good" or "bad" nutrient is less than helpful. And, as Marion Nestle points out, "the context of the lifestyle matters, too."[1]

In his book *Outliers*, Malcolm Gladwell tells the story of an Italian community that, despite having relatively high rates of overweight citizens and diets rich in all the things that are supposed to be bad for you, had no heart disease to speak of.[2] Researchers were intrigued by what they regarded as a puzzle, eventually figuring out that the low stress and highly interactive nature of their community life was the factor that kept them healthy. Gladwell's interest is less in diet and lifestyle than in the unexamined factors that contribute to success and well-being, but I can't help but see that this story confirms the truth of Nestle's contention that we can't separate nutrients from foods, foods from diets, and diets from lifestyles. Everything is important, even (and maybe especially) the things we don't think matter much at all.

Like *joy*.

As we've seen thus far, eating with joy is more than simply sitting down and enjoying your food (although that's a big part of it!). Eating with joy means accepting food as God's gift—"God's love made edible," as Norman Wirzba put it.[3] It means choosing food, as far as we are able, that affirms a flourishing life for the land, for the animals and for the people that bring us our food. It means eating food with others in ways that lead to our mutual health and flourishing. And it means embracing our creativity as people made in the image of the Creator God to prepare food in ways that celebrate God's gift while bringing enjoyment to all our senses.

GRATEFUL PERMISSIVENESS

Today France is a largely secular society; their national "religion" is cuisine. Much as American evangelicals might debate arcane points of theology or argue about the nature of the Communion elements or get into conflicts over hymns versus choruses, in France people argue about the proper proportions of butter to flour in a béchamel sauce, whether a *Gratin Dauphinois* is made with cheese or not, and which region produces the best beef, cheese, butter or wine. But more than that, preparing food with creativity and care, eating together, savoring each bite and relaxing with a glass of something are pursued with religious fervor. It's all these things, in combination with the broader French lifestyle that includes lots of walking, cycling and time outdoors— not the isolated resverotrols found in red wine—that lead to lower levels of heart disease and cancer.

I'm not suggesting that we all move to France, or even that we attempt to "be more French" in the ways we eat. But France's food culture certainly has some lessons for us, lessons in slowing down, observing the seasons, appreciating the bounty of local "food-sheds," eating with others and eating with enjoyment. (Remember the bestselling book *French Women Don't Get Fat?* That's not true, of course, but the subtitle says it all: *The Secret of Eating for Pleasure.*) Perhaps best of all, in France (and Europe more generally) the national food culture is not widely perceived as a concern of wealthy, fussy gourmets. Not at all! Everyone *has* to eat, but "food as fuel" is not even a consideration. In France, food is love, food is celebration, food is delicious. In this context, praise and thanks to the God who makes all this bounty and enjoyment possible seems only natural.

A joyful food culture is at odds with the various restrictive diets that are continually making their rounds in the news, on bookshelves and in people's minds. Almost without exception, diets in all their variety share the distinction of making it difficult to eat with others, difficult to eat what's at hand and difficult to enjoy what you're eating. Moreover, the restrictive attitude that comes with dieting (some things are "allowed," some are "forbidden," some are "good," some are "bad") seems itself to call forth from people the "Eden syndrome"—we start to crave the one thing we're not allowed to have, which is why again and again diets have been found to be woefully ineffective at sustaining long-term change of *any* kind. In *Seeking the Straight and Narrow*, Lynne Gerber notes that participants in the popular program First Place found that doing the "calorie reports" was unhelpful and "a distraction from the main purpose of the program: focusing more on God and less on food."[4] According to Ellyn Satter, adults who are comfortable enjoying food in satisfying amounts—explicitly *rejecting* a restrictive attitude toward food—are more likely to remain at a healthy weight and have healthier "numbers" (like cholesterol and blood pressure) than those who aren't. It's paradoxical, but it makes sense: when you make all things permissible, you're able to enjoy yourself without guilt and anxiety.

So eat with the joy that comes from sincere gratitude to the God who brings forth food from the earth! When you are a guest at someone else's table, when you are in a place where a packet of peanut butter crackers is your best "meal" option, when you are eating at home by yourself, you are in the presence of God. Whatever the fare, it is from God. So thank God. Enjoy his provision!

LETTING FOOD SPEAK OF GOD'S GOODNESS IN PROCURING AND PREPARING

Not all food speaks of God's goodness with equal clarity. There are foods, like chocolate and coffee, for example, that come to us too often through the pain and suffering of other human beings. An estimated 200,000 children are enslaved on cocoa plantations on the west coast of Africa, while countless farmers who produce items like coffee, vanilla, palm oil, sugar and coconut struggle to get by on what they can earn for their labor.

Fair trade may not be a perfect fix to the injustices suffered by these people in the Majority World, but it is for certain a big step in the right direction. While you will certainly pay more for fair trade products, you are also tangibly *loving your neighbor* through your responsible choices. It's also worth considering the money you spend on fair trade foods as a form of aid. The international poverty and justice advocacy organization Oxfam estimates that for every dollar the developed world gives in aid, it *takes away* two dollars *through unfair trade.* This doesn't mean that you can do away with child sponsorship if you're drinking fair trade coffee, but it *does* mean that it's worth considering whether those candy-bar fundraising efforts for charity aren't at cross-purposes. When you consider that most of these imported items are *luxuries*—not necessities—it seems (at least to me) all the more imperative to make every effort to purchase the fairly traded variety. Voluntarily avoiding foods that are known to come to us via the suffering of others is a small sacrifice to make for the sake of loving God and our neighbors.

Chocolate, coffee and other imported luxuries, however, are *not* the only foods whose production has an impact on our neighbors. Highly processed foods—like fast food—are destructive to people's health, cruel to animals and damaging to God's creation, in large part due to the government subsidies of crops like corn, soy and wheat (which also create unfair trade relationships with other nations by flooding world markets with cheap grain). A meal from McDonald's can't speak clearly of God's love and provision for creatures because of the many, many injustices involved at every stage of its production. In contrast, by purchasing and preparing fresh foods from the best sources available to you, you can allow the food that graces your plate and nourishes your body to speak more clearly of the sustaining hand of God, which turns the days and seasons and, with the help of people, coaxes food from the earth—a beautiful thing. Yet at the same time, I would say that for the sake of love, better the occasional meal shared with friends at McDonald's than organic salad in bitter isolation.

The best place to start is at home. If you have any outdoor space at all—even if it's only a roof top or a small plot in a community garden—you can grow some of your own food. Obviously, this book can't be a manual on all the necessary arts, but I would encourage you to grow *something*, even if it's just some edible herbs in a window box. Some vegetables are tricky to grow (I never have managed to get a good head on my broccoli), but others, like broccoli raab and string beans, spring from the earth with very little encouragement. As Wendell Berry says, a vegetable garden solves several problems while creating no new ones (other than what to do with all that zucchini).[5] When you grow your own food, you know for certain how it was grown and by whom! There is no danger that the vegetables have been treated with something you don't want your kids eating, and they do not have to travel long distances by truck to get to you.

There are other reasons to garden: it is great exercise, it gives you respect for people who have to grow *all* their own food (it can be hard!) and it tunes you in to the created world. There are few places I feel the presence of God—and profound gratitude to him—more fully than in my vegetable garden. It's a place where I can think, get some exercise and spend time in the sunshine and fresh air. It's a place where I can contemplate the mystery of an eight-foot-tall giant of a tomato plant coming from a seed so tiny that twenty of them could fit on a dime—and the reality of my persistent doubt that something so puny-looking would ever amount to anything. It's a place where I experience delight in watching the gradual ripening of the first spring strawberries and the exuberance of our children over the first spicy red radishes popping from the earth.

Gardening does take time and space and know-how, and not everyone has those things. In recent years, CSA (community supported agriculture) programs have become extremely popular. When you join a CSA, you pay the farmers in advance for a share of their crops. Some CSAs are produce-only, but many include milk, eggs, meat, poultry and even honey; and usually you have the option to choose what things you want to include in your share. It can take a little Internet-sleuthing and asking around, but chances are, wherever you live, you will be able to find a relatively local source for at least some of your food. And the advantages here, as with gardening, are that you can get to know where your food comes from in a more intimate way, make connections with the people and animals whose labor feeds you, and in so doing, give thanks to God with greater understanding of what you're thanking him for! For me, cracking open the eggs I buy from a neighbor with a backyard chicken coop is a totally different experience than cracking open grocery store eggs. I thank God for both kinds of eggs, but with the first kind, I can thank God for *Stacey's* eggs and in my mind see those silly hens poking around in the grass for grubs.

It's true that choosing local and responsibly raised foods can, like fairly traded foods, cost more money. If I compare a box of organic cookies with a box of Chips Ahoy, the price difference is particularly upsetting! But when you make an effort to reduce the amount of packaged foods (chips, crackers, cookies) with fresh or homemade things—you may just find that your food bill doesn't increase so much. Of course, the flip side of *that* is that unprocessed foods have to be processed—by *you!* As a homeschooling, work-at-home mom, I know that time is precious and that cooking takes time. But I also know that advertisers have been trying to convince us all since at least the 1950s that cooking is *hard*, that it takes *too much time* and that we're all *too busy* to do it. Truth to tell, most of the meals I cook take less than an hour to prepare, and many of our mainstay meals can be prepared in thirty minutes or less. And, if we're honest with ourselves, we could probably make the time to cook *something* sometime in the day. After all, we've made time for the Internet, for apps and for watching the cooking shows that have, ironically, burgeoned in popularity in recent years even as home cooking has declined. Making a simple dish of pasta with sauce and vegetables more or less from scratch can easily take less time than watching *Rachael Ray*.

What if we choose to view cooking as a creative act instead of drudgery? What if we use the time chopping, cutting, sautéing and steaming to take in the sights, smells, sounds, textures and tastes of the food we are preparing? For me, practicing mindfulness while cooking is another way of experiencing God's creation while exercising my own creativity. I love to chop onions in perfect dice and then toss them into a hot pan with olive oil, watching as they release steam and slowly turn translucent and finally caramelize into a rich brown, ready to form the basis for everything from chili to spicy peanut sauce to beef stew. And that's just the onions! As I cook, tasting as I go, making mental note of what's in the refrigerator, cupboards and garden, I'm inspired to experiment a bit—Would a pinch of paprika give that a bit more bite? Would a dab of butter improve the texture?—and create a bit of everyday culture. It's not to say that I never tire of cooking. I certainly do, and once-weekly Chinese takeout is our family ritual. But most of the time, the creative energy I get from cooking replenishes rather than drains me. Maybe that has come with time and practice; I don't know for sure. But I do know that many, many people find satisfaction in learning to prepare food simply and well.

SIMPLICITY AND CELEBRATION

The words *simplicity* and *celebration*—or, if you like, "ferial" (ordinary) and "festal" (feast day)—are helpful in shaping a practice of joyful eating day to day, week to week, year by year. The alternating rhythms of feast days and ordinary days belong to the church year and to cultures that still follow traditional and seasonal patterns of eating, but this is a cycle that most of us have all but lost. In some of my favorite children's books, the Little House series, it's clear that the festal/ferial rhythm was still very much in play in their pioneer family. Most days, meals were fairly simple, sugar was used sparingly, and the store-bought kind was reserved for company. But Christmas, for example, called for several kinds of meat, numerous rich side dishes, and all sorts of homemade pies, cookies and candies. The Ingalls family's consumption was so simple that a Christmas on which they were given a peppermint stick, hand-knit mittens and a homemade ragdoll was a "very rich Christmas" indeed. In the *More-with-Less* cookbook, Doris Janzen Longacre describes the ratcheting-up effect of consumption in terms of cake frosting:

> My grandmother iced cakes only for birthdays. My mother iced most of her cakes, but thinly and only between the layers and on top—not on the sides. Until recently, I stirred up an ample bowlful of frosting that covered everything and left plenty of finger-lickin's.

If we feast every day, we have to *really* go overboard to make special days "special." Better, to my mind, is an intentional simplicity for the ordinary days so that special days can be given their due.

Often, I think, people respond to overconsumption with well-intentioned austerity diets that leave very little room for celebration. Cupcakes might not be everyday foods, but that doesn't mean your kids shouldn't have them to celebrate birthdays! Intentionally simplifying our eating on "ordinary days" makes room for greater joy on the days that we want to mark as special. We don't eat desserts most days, which heightens the uniqueness and specialness of birthdays, when we eat cake. Because we eat a lot of simple foods—beans and rice, vegetarian stews, soup and bread—a nice beef stew can be a celebration meal. It's actually freeing to orient yourself toward a festal-ferial approach to food. It frees you from feeling that every eating occasion must be celebration-worthy, and it frees you to exercise your culinary creativity for days of true celebration.[6]

In addition to gratitude—perhaps as an accessory to gratitude—cultivating the virtue of slowness is crucial to a practice of joyful eating. We live in a food culture that values *speed* above almost everything. I can't tell you how many meals I have rushed through in order to get through them and back to whatever other, more "important" thing I was doing. When I was a driven young college student, I felt virtuous for skipping cafeteria meals or getting by with a yogurt drink that I'd gulp in the hallway between classes. I've even rushed through dessert! But rushing through food doesn't make joyful eating very easy. It isn't conducive to cultivating a keen awareness of food as God's gracious and delicious provision. It doesn't respect the care and creativity that, at every step, brought the food to us. Cooks often complain about how fast everyone eats at the dinner table, even on Thanksgiving. ("Why even bother cooking a nice meal if everyone's going to be done eating in fifteen minutes?") Slowing down, paying attention to the food and to the people who made it and with whom we're eating allows us to take in more deeply the pleasures of the table, made possible by the hand of the God who feeds us all.[7]

All of these suggestions for putting a joyful kind of eating into practice are, as you might have guessed, best pursued in community—and *that's* not always easy. It can be hard to get a spouse or children excited about making changes in the way you eat. And yet, as I've highlighted throughout the book, eating is a profoundly social act. It would be difficult to overemphasize the importance of making time to eat with other people. For all the many criti-

cisms I have of weight-loss programs, the truth is, there is a lot of
wisdom in gathering people into groups to further common goals.
But joining together to *diet* isn't what I have in mind. I have in
mind something like Slow Food *convivia*—regular gatherings of
people who want to enjoy good, simple food in one another's
company. A Mennonite church I visited in Chicago had soup and
bread after services on Sunday. The soups and breads would vary,
but for the sake of simplicity, it was always soup and bread. It's
well documented that meals together are beneficial to people's
health; eating with others is a natural appetite regulator. It is also
an occasion to commune with one another on equal terms—to
acknowledge our shared humanity and to enjoy God's gifts in an
incarnated way. These two concepts—*eating together* with *gratitude toward God*—are the heart of joyful eating.

REDEMPTIVE MOVEMENT AND SYMBOLIC ACTS

Sometimes, despite my high ideals and aspirations always to
practice joyful eating before God and with love for my neighbor, I
find myself in situations where the best I can do is far less than
"perfect." Sometimes I eat a hastily slapped together sandwich
while I'm running out the door, forgetting even to taste it, much
less to thank God for it. Sometimes I find myself eating at a restaurant with friends, or at the home of someone who doesn't share
any of my convictions about food and eating. Sometimes people
offer my kids snacks that I would never choose for them. How do
I negotiate these situations, and how do they fit into a life of practicing joyful eating?

I try my best not to stand in judgment of the food that someone
else serves me.[8] Even though I've spent several years writing
mainly about food, I'm a Christian first; and as strongly as I feel
about food as a conduit of God's love and as a site for loving God
and neighbor, choosing the "right" kind of food (whatever that is)
is much less important to me than giving thanks to God and being

kind to my neighbor. I feel it would be an unkindness to refuse something that has been offered to me in fellowship and in love for the sake of my convictions about food. While it's not exactly equivalent, I think of Paul's exhortation to Peter to eat with Gentiles for the sake of the gospel and of Christian fellowship, even though that was counter to his deeply embedded cultural preferences. My friend John Edwards, who has been for many years a missionary in Japan, notes that he can always tell right away which American interns will go far in Japanese ministries: they're the ones who are most willing to *try* some of the stranger foods offered to them by their Japanese hosts. I think it's important to keep in mind the possibility that food preferences—even ones made on ethical grounds—are seldom a good reason to insult a host or impede fellowship.

I also think it's important to realize that *none* of us get it (and by "it" I mean "everything") right all the time. Facing that reality can cause us to want to stop trying completely. My mother is an enthusiastic and passionate person who tends to get carried away when she encounters new ideas or practices. Once, she gave up sugar "forever" and threw out everything in the house that had sugar in it, even the ketchup and Worcestershire sauce. It wasn't long before she grew frustrated with this restrictive plan and made a late-night run for a pint of Häagen-Dazs, which I found her eating straight from the carton. Another time, after reading one of Michael Pollan's books, she became so obsessed with eating "real food" and so worried about what was or was not real food that she ended up not getting enough to eat, until she was so hungry that she gobbled several hotdogs at her school's field day. Extreme practices, such as those attempted by "No Impact Man," make for good publicity, but for most people, they don't represent a workable lifestyle. Returning to low-impact local patterns of consumption will work well for some people in some places, but many folks can't dedicate the amount of time and effort that a perfectly local and sustainable diet requires.

But the perfect need never be the enemy of the good. In a very different book challenging overly simplistic Bible application, New Testament scholar William Webb points out that God's commands to people—such as the purity laws in Leviticus, and even some of the specific prescriptions of Paul within the epistles—do not necessarily represent the real-world "ideal" God has.[9] Rather, God moves *redemptively*, starting with where people are in time and place and moving them incrementally closer to God's ideal. The law that a rapist must marry his victim seems crazy, even cruel to us, but within the culture of the ancient Near East, it made sense and was, in fact, redemptive: a rape victim would be worse off than a murder victim because in that culture, no one would marry her. What we have in the concrete-specific ("surface") meaning of Scripture, says Webb, doesn't necessarily represent God's perfect "as it is in heaven" will for all time. Most North American Christian men don't greet one another with a "holy kiss." That was appropriate in that cultural context, but isn't in ours. We find other ways to extend a warm and loving welcome to people.

What this has to do with joyful eating is much simpler: it's best to accept that you are never going to do it all right. Aiming for "perfection" (whatever that might be) is a recipe for frustration (Eccles 7). It is best to start where you are and aim to *move redemptively*. Your family doesn't eat together much? Don't suddenly announce that every meal of every day will be eaten together or else! Instead, slowly and incrementally work your way up to more shared meals. You never cook? Don't toss out all the take-out menus, but don't toss out your cookbooks either. Start with one or two meals a week and work toward an ideal that's reasonable for you. Not sure you can afford local and organic produce? Try planning just one local meal a week and go from there. Start where you are. *Practice.*

As Doris Janzen Longacre writes in the first part of her cookbook/manifesto *More-with-Less*:

> As Christians dealing with human hurts, we have to remind ourselves again and again that we are not called to be successful, but to be faithful. Our first directions come from the way Jesus told us to live, not from what we think will work.[10]

Someone might protest that if food choices are ethically significant, if they matter in how people and animals are treated and if they matter to God, how can incremental steps make a difference? Don't we need to go *all the way*? But even if we do go all the way, will one family's choices really matter in the global scale of things?

Individuals making small incremental changes can, slowly change a whole food culture. Don't discount the real effects of your choices, even small ones. But *even if* the choices you make to eat with joy are only symbolic (which I'm not sure they are), they are still worth pursuing. Years ago now, when I was in the early stages of my own journey toward eating with joy, I listened to a lecture by N. T. Wright, the former Anglican bishop of Durham, at Regent College in Vancouver. At the time I was struggling with how to handle the weight of the world's food problems on my shoulders, wondering things like: *Is it wrong for me to buy "luxuries" like coffee when so many don't even have clean water? Will reducing my meat consumption—and consumption in general—really make the lives of other people in other places appreciably better? Is this just something I'm doing to make* myself *feel better?*

And then I heard N. T. Wright say this:

> *Don't despise the small but significant symbolic act.* We live still in this modernist dream which says, "Unless you can change the whole thing, it's not even worth trying." That's not what Jesus did. Jesus did small but significant symbolic acts, each one of which was freighted with kingdom meaning. *God probably doesn't want you to reorganize [everything] over-*

night—learn to be symbol-makers and storytellers for the kingdom. Learn to model genuine humanness in your worship and your stewardship and your relationships—the Church's task vis-à-vis the world is to model true humanness as a sign, as an invitation.[11]

Resist the temptation to think that if you can't change the whole system, it's not worth doing anything. Moving redemptively toward joyful eating as best we can—the kind that most fully speaks of God's kingdom of peace and justice and abundant good taste—may be all we can do.

Shaping a different food culture—a joyful, healthy, flourishing and tasty food culture, where humans can be more fully human, animals and plants can be more fully themselves, and God can be more fully enjoyed in our cultivating, creating and sharing; indeed, realizing the Supper of the Lamb—this doesn't happen overnight.

It happens bite by bite: "Give us *this day* our daily bread . . . "

So go and *eat with joy!*

PRAYERS BEFORE MEALS

Blessed God, who gives food to all creatures,
fill our hearts with joy and gladness, that we
may abound in every good work in Christ
Jesus our Lord; with whom to you be glory,
honor and might, with the Holy Spirit: one
God, now and forever. Amen.

Adapted from an Egyptian monastic blessing

We cannot love you, God, unless we love each other,
And to love each other we must know each other in the breaking of bread—
As the disciples knew Christ after the resurrection.

Here, at this table, we are not alone—you are with us as we are
with one another.
Heaven is a banquet, and life is a banquet, too,
Even with only a dry crust shared in companionship.
Love comes with community.
Bless this food
Bless us as we love one another, and as we love You.
Amen.

Adapted by Rachel Stone from a quote from Dorothy Day

Lord Jesus, be our holy guest,
Our morning joy, our evening rest,
And with our daily bread impart,
Your love and peace to every heart.
Amen.

RECILES

RECIPES

Peppermint Bark

Nourishing? Depends on your definition, I guess. This treat is
easy and fun to make. Once, when my son was down in the dumps,
making up a batch of this stuff really cheered him up—probably
partly because I let him break the candy canes up with a hammer
(after they'd been sealed in a bag, of course). A very small piece for
everyone, enjoyed slowly after dinner, is a sweet way to end a meal
together. Please consider using organic and fair-trade ingredients
if possible, and count the extra cost as bringing sweetness—not
bitterness—to the lives of the people who brought it to you.

First, break **6 regular-sized peppermint candy canes** into
lentil-sized fragments, either putting them in a sealed bag and
striking with a wooden mallet or whirling them quickly in a food
processor. (Smashing is much more fun.) Melt **18 ounces white
chocolate** in a glass bowl in the microwave or in a double boiler.

On a baking sheet lined with waxed paper, draw a rectangle with a pencil. Pour **2/3 cup (about half) of the melted white chocolate** in the center of the rectangle, and quickly spread the chocolate evenly to all the edges. Sprinkle immediately with about **1/2 the candy canes** and let rest for 10 minutes. Meanwhile, melt **9 ounces semisweet chocolate.** Stir in **1 1/2 teaspoons pure peppermint extract and 6 tablespoons heavy cream.** When you are sure that the first layer of white chocolate is hardened, pour the semisweet-cream mixture evenly over that first layer and allow to harden—about 20 minutes. Rewarm the white chocolate and spread over the semisweet layer, sprinkling the white chocolate with the rest of the crushed candy canes. When fully hardened, use a sharp knife to cut the bark into one-inch square pieces. Store in an airtight container with layers of wax paper in between them, or pack into empty glass jam jars and share the minty goodness.

Peppermint bark makes a fun present. Make sure that the recipient tastes it while it's still nice and fresh, ideally within the first three days and certainly within the week.

Orzo Summer Salad
This is just the thing for a hot summer night. It's cool and delicious and uses lots of seasonal produce. Pasta salads are almost always best eaten the day they're made, but in our experience this one lasts nicely for a day or two. It's great packed in a cooler and eaten at a picnic.

First, prepare the dressing:
2 tablespoons freshly squeezed lemon juice
1 tablespoon red wine vinegar
3 tablespoons olive oil
1/2 teaspoon each freshly ground black pepper and salt
1/2 teaspoon minced garlic

Set aside.

Meanwhile, cook **1 cup uncooked orzo** according to package directions, subtracting 2 minutes from the suggested cooking time. (You want it a little *al dente*.) Rinse in cold water and drain, placing in a large bowl. Stir in a bit of the dressing to keep the orzo from getting clumpy.

Add:

1-2 cups chopped, seeded tomato (or equivalent halved cherry or grape tomatoes)

1 cup cubed fresh mozzarella or feta cheese

1/4 cup chopped fresh basil

1/2 cup finely diced red onion

2 cups corn kernels, sliced off the cob and quickly sautéed, then cooled

Mix the vegetables and cheese with the orzo and pour on the rest of the dressing. Mix well and chill in refrigerator for half an hour or so before serving. Delicious!

• •

POINTS FOR ACTION

- Aim for simplicity. Soup and bread is a good lunch or dinner. Remember, celebrations can be made special by aiming for simplicity the rest of the time.

- Avoid "nutritionism," the idea that the goodness of a food comes from its constituent parts or that the only point of eating is to confer health.

- If your church or small group doesn't regularly practice sharing food together, try to make that happen, even if it is a simple breaking of bread—or veggie sticks and dip.

- Join your local chapter of Slow Food and participate in the *convivia* potlucks. You'll meet other people interested in good food and you'll learn a lot. Or start your own group!

- Consider the assumptions behind your various patterns of food consumption. Are there times of the day when you eat mindlessly? Do you graze? You might try "eating the hours" (a practice described by J. Brent Bill in *Awaken Your Senses*) or otherwise orienting your eating toward a more mindful practice.

- Make incremental goals. Not long ago a friend told me of his plans to go vegan for the sake of his Type 1 diabetes. I told him, "Great—but don't go back to eating at McDonald's and drinking 32-ounce sodas because veganism is too restrictive!" Slow and steady is preferable to all-or-nothing.

- Move redemptively and joyfully. Joy is subversive!

For Further Reading

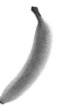

On Eating and Theology

Capon, Robert Farrar. *The Supper of the Lamb: A Culinary Reflection*. New York: Modern Library, 2002.

Fields, Leslie Leyland, ed. *The Spirit of Food: 34 Writers on Feasting and Fasting Toward God*. Eugene, OR: Wipf & Stock, 2010.

Miles, Sara. *Take This Bread: A Radical Conversion*. New York: Ballantine Books, 2008.

Wirzba, Norman. *Food and Faith: A Theology of Eating*. New York: Cambridge University Press, 2011.

On Eating and Justice

Ehrenreich, Barbara. *Nickel and Dimed: On (Not) Getting By in America*. New York: Picador, 2011.

McMillan, Tracie. *The American Way of Eating: Undercover at Walmart, Applebee's, Farm Fields and the Dinner Table*. New York: Scribner, 2012.

Nestle, Marion. *Food Politics: How the Food Industry Influences Nutrition and Health*. California Studies in Food and Culture. 2nd rev. ed. Berkeley: University of California Press, 2007.

Schut, Michael, ed. *Food and Faith: Justice, Joy, and Daily Bread*. New York: Morehouse Publishing, 2010.

Simon, Michelle. *Appetite for Profit: How the Food Industry Undermines Our Health and How to Fight Back*. New York: Nation Books, 2006.

On Eating Together

Brown, Harriet. *Brave Girl Eating: A Family's Struggle with Anorexia.* New York: William Morrow, 2010.

Capon, Robert Farrar. *Party Spirit: Some Entertaining Principles.* New York: William Morrow, 1979 (out of print).

Collins, Laura. *Eating with Your Anorexic: How My Child Recovered Through Family-Based Treatment and Yours Can Too.* New York: McGraw-Hill, 2004.

David, Laurie, and Kirstin Uhrenholdt. *The Family Dinner: Great Ways to Connect with Your Kids, One Meal at a Time.* New York: Grand Central Life & Style, 2010.

Weinstein, Miriam. *The Surprising Power of Family Meals: How Eating Together Makes Us Smarter, Stronger, Healthier and Happier.* Hanover, NH: Steerforth Books, 2006.

On Eating Sustainably

Bahnson, Fred, and Norman Wirzba. *Making Peace with the Land: God's Call to Reconcile with Creation.* Resources for Reconciliation. Downers Grove, IL: InterVarsity Press, 2012.

Berry, Wendell. *The Unsettling of America: Culture & Agriculture.* San Francisco: Sierra Club Books, 1996.

Kingsolver, Barbara, with Steven Hopp and Camille Kingsolver. *Animal, Vegetable, Miracle: A Year of Food Life.* New York: Harper Perennial, 2008.

Pollan, Michael. *The Omnivore's Dilemma: A Natural History of Four Meals.* New York: Penguin, 2006.

———. *In Defense of Food: An Eater's Manifesto.* New York: Penguin, 2009.

On Eating Creatively

Allen, John S. *The Omnivorous Mind: Our Evolving Relationship with Food.* Boston: Harvard University Press, 2012.

Bill, J. Brent, and Beth Booram. *Awaken Your Senses: Exercises for Exploring the Wonder of God.* Downers Grove, IL: InterVarsity Press, 2012.

McGee, Harold. *On Food and Cooking: The Science and Lore of the Kitchen.* New York: Scribner, 2004.

Ruhlman, Michael. *The Making of a Chef: Mastering Heat at the Culinary Institute of America.* New York: Holt Paperbacks, 2009.

On Cooking

Bauer, Elise. *Simply Recipes blog,* May 2, 2012, http://simplyrecipes .com.

Bittman, Mark. *The Food Matters Cookbook: 500 Revolutionary Recipes for Better Living.* New York: Simon & Schuster, 2010.

Editors at Cook's Illustrated. *The Cook's Illustrated Cookbook: 2,000 Recipes from 20 Years of America's Most Trusted Cooking Magazine.* 2011.

Hockman-Wert, Cathleen, and Mary Beth Lind. *Simply in Season.* Expanded ed. World Community Cookbook. Scottdale, PA: Herald Press, 2009.

Longacre, Doris Janzen. *The More-with-Less Cookbook.* 25th anniv. ed. A World Community Cookbook. Scottdale, PA: Herald Press, 2010.

On Eating/Body Image Issues

Satter, Ellyn. *Secrets of Feeding a Healthy Family: How to Eat, How to Raise Healthy Eaters, How to Cook.* 2nd ed. Madison, WI: Kelcy Press, 2008.

Tribole, Evelyn, and Elyse Resch. *Intuitive Eating: A Revolutionary Program That Works.* New York: St. Martin's Griffen, 2003.

Group Discussion Guide

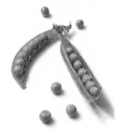

You may plan to meet several times, discussing one or two chapters each time, or meet once and discuss the whole book in one go. Either way, why not plan on eating together—perhaps trying some recipes from the book—as part of your time together?

INTRODUCTION: Conflicted Eating
and
CHAPTER 1: Joyful Eating

1. When you think of food, what issues, problems or struggles come to mind?

2. Can you relate to what the author shares of her story? How is your story similar to or different from hers?

3. The author says that "God made eating sustaining, delicious and pleasurable because God is all those things and more." How do you respond to this statement?

4. Had you previously noticed the role that food plays in Scripture? How do contemporary Westerners interact with food differently than people in biblical times?

5. What is your reaction to the author's claim that God wants to feed us like a "nursing mother"? How have cultural assumptions (about God and breasts!) made that image one that people struggle with?

6. If you are a parent, what does the metaphor of God as feeding parent say to you? Do you find yourself troubled by the story of Holly (the baby who was made to feel shame for her pleasure in eating)?

7. "Jesus as 'Bread of Heaven' is spiritual truth, but also living metaphor." What does this mean? How might we receive food as a metaphor of Christ's love?

Suggestion: Plan a time to view and discuss *Babette's Feast* with your reading group.

CHAPTER 2: Generous Eating

1. Think of a time you encountered someone who was not getting enough to eat. How did you respond?

2. What assumptions do you have regarding the eating habits of people who are poor? Were they challenged by this chapter?

3. Have you experienced a church or Christian community that came close to the ideals of table fellowship expressed in the early church?

4. What do you think of the author's claim that diet-related diseases are as much the fault of corporations as they are of individuals?

5. How do you see the passage from Amos 8:5-6 relating to the contemporary food landscape?

6. What goes through your mind when you read something like "Even people who have never heard the name of Jesus know the name of Coke"?

7. How do we balance individual responses (eating less fast food) with larger, system-wide responses (ending unfair subsidies)? Why are both important?

Suggestion: Your group could gather to watch *Fast Food Nation* or PBS's Exposé "20,000 Cuts a Day."

CHAPTER 3: Communal Eating

1. When do you tend to eat alone, and when do you eat with others? Describe how eating with others figures (or doesn't figure) into your life.

2. What are the benefits and drawbacks of eating alone verus eating together?

3. How was eating together important and significant in the early church?

4. Have you experienced the decline of the family meal in your lifetime? What effects do you think the decline of family meals has?

5. How do food allergies, preferences and diets impede communal eating? What are some ways we can bridge differences to encourage communal eating in spite of differences?

6. The author describes taking meals to a friend in the nursing home and establishing a regular routine of church potlucks. What are some other ways of using food to minister to people?

7. What are some of the obstacles to hospitality in your life? What are some simple steps you could take to eat more meals with others?

   Suggestion: Watch *Mostly Martha* as a group.

CHAPTER 4: Restorative Eating

1. This chapter discusses eating disorders. How have eating disorders been a part of your experience—or that of people close to you?

2. What are some of the cultural factors influencing high rates of disorder and poor self-image when it comes to bodies?

3. Discuss the social isolation of anorexics described in the chapter. What might influence and exacerbate this isolation?

4. Have you heard of family-based treatment? How might the lessons of family-based treatment inform "ordinary" eating practices of a family?

5. How is "solitary eating" problematic? How does this chapter relate to the previous one in this regard?

6. How might eating be more restorative and healing in the lives of those around you?

Suggestion: You might consider watching the documentary *Thin* by Lauren Greenfield. Be advised, the film might be a trigger to those struggling with eating disorders. If you watch it, be sure to critique the treatment style of the Renfrew center.

CHAPTER 5: Sustainable Eating

1. Describe a memory you have of gardening or visiting a farm. What was it like to see where food comes from?

2. Have you experienced Christian skepticism of climate crisis, or is that a thing of the past?

3. How does Scripture invite us to celebrate and respect God's creation?

4. Is there a balance in regarding ourselves as co-creatures with animals and sovereigns over creation?

5. Discuss the very different stories of two Nobel laureates, Fritz Haber and Wangari Maathai, and their very different views of nature.

6. The author spends a good bit of time talking about biodiversity. What is it, what endangers it, and why does it matter?

7. What changes in your diet are you considering after reading this chapter? What changes have you already made (perhaps prior to reading the book) and why?

Suggestion: Watch the documentary film *Food, Inc.* as a group.

CHAPTER 6: Creative Eating

1. What's your favorite food or meal to make? Why?
2. What are some different food cultures you've experienced? How do they differ, and how do they assume different things about the world?
3. How is food culture related to culture making more broadly?
4. Have you experienced a culture of suspicion of pleasure in food? How has that taken shape? What does Robert Farrar Capon mean when he says calories are "idols"?
5. How have you experienced cooking as creative or uncreative?
6. Does inexpensive and readily available prepared food discourage you from cooking?
7. What are the reasons the author gives for pursuing cooking as culture making?
8. In what ways might your meals become culture-making activities for your family, church or community?

Suggestion: Watch the Disney/Pixar movie *Ratatouille* and discuss in light of this chapter. Or plan to prepare and eat a meal together.

CHAPTER 7: Redemptive Eating

1. The author describes how people often assume she's about to judge their dietary habits. Have you experienced dietary judgmentalism? What forms does it take?
2. Marion Nestle is quoted as saying, "The problem with nutrient-by-nutrient science is that it *takes the nutrient out of the context of the food, the food out of the context of the diet, and the diet out of the context of the lifestyle*" (emphasis added). Discuss what this might mean in light of the broader concept of joyful eating.

3. How does restriction foster rebellion?

4. The author discusses adopting a festal/ferial approach to food, as well as the "ratcheting up" effect of culture where abundance is sometimes simply *too much*. How might a festal/ferial approach work differently than, say, a diet mentality?

5. Discuss the concept of redemptive movement as it relates to joyful eating in the book and in your own life.

6. The author writes, "choosing the 'right' kind of food (whatever that is) is much less important to me than giving thanks to God and being kind to my neighbor." How is that different from or similar to your own perspective?

7. Does the "small symbolic act" have significance? Why or why not?

8. What might you do to help others eat more redemptively?

Suggestion: Close your reading group with a shared meal, or plan to meet again in a few months for a meal to share your own stories of joyful eating.

Acknowledgments

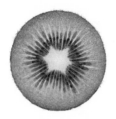

Mrs. Charlotte Rich, my kindergarten teacher at P.S. 222 in Brooklyn, New York, helped me learn to read and write and was the first of many good teachers who nurtured my love of words. I am thankful to my many teachers for their encouragement and instruction over the years, but especially to Denise Hayden, RoseLee Bancroft, Brian Toews, Allen Frantzen and the late Samuel Hsu. The staff at the Floyd Memorial Library have been my faithful teachers as well. Thank you for your patience with my endless interlibrary loan piles and the miles of printouts you've endured so I could get the materials I needed.

The journey to publication is seldom straight, and I am thankful to so many people who helped along the way: Kendra Langdon Juskus and Rusty Pritchard, who helped me hone my first-ever published articles; Sarah Pulliam Bailey and Katelyn Beaty who welcomed me at the *Christianity Today* women's blog, and so many others. Andy McGuire at Bethany House expressed enthusiasm for this project and advised me to start blogging (which I did—thanks, Andy!); Chris Park of Foundry Media and Amy Julia Becker helped me connect with Al Hsu at IVP, who has, at every point, been full of grace, wisdom and good humor. He is the perfect editor for this project. I am honored and humbled to work with the team at IVP: people who love God with their hearts, souls, minds and strength. Thank you.

I am grateful for the friends who have provided insight as well as companionship along the journey: Kristin Egan and Marietta Liebengood read huge portions of the book in close to its present state; Adriel Driver read it in its more nascent form. Danielle Matava and Nicki Wilkins, in our St. Andrews "story group," lent me their ears for more than a few evenings. As a fellow writer, Ellen Painter Dollar has offered her keen insight and warm friendship. Margaret Kim Peterson and Amy Frykholm, both of whom I met late in the birth of this book, have been sources of wisdom, inspiration and friendship.

This book could not have been written without my family. Shari Franco, my godmother, and Sarah Gutierrez, my godsister (it's not a word, but should be), have shared countless meals, games and conversations. You have encouraged me with your faithfulness more than you know. I have written this book in large part for you and in honor of Grandma Donna, with whom we all shared many slices of chocolate cake with sides of calorie anxiety. May we, and she, rest in the amazing grace of the God who loves to feed us all.

My dad, Tom LaMothe, is always up for a late night beer-and-bull session. If it weren't for his Irish parenting, I would have quit everything every time anything felt too hard. My mom, Jeanette, helped care for my boys so I could write; but more than that, she has been my faithful friend. Both my parents have given me grace, for which I am profoundly grateful.

Aidan and Graeme, it's when we sit and eat together—and you tell me your stories and your ideas and plans—that I feel most at home. It was in watching God bring forth your bodies from mine that I found healing and wholeness. Thank you for your patience (most of the time!) with my long hours in front of my computer.

Tim, without you this book would never have come to be. Your love has opened me to myself, to the world, to our God. You are an *'ish gabor chayil.*

Notes

Introduction: Conflicted Eating

[1]Lynne Gerber, *Seeking the Straight and Narrow* (Chicago: University of Chicago Press, 2012), p. 192.

[2]See my review of Gerber's book in *The Christian Century* (forthcoming).

[3]See Lyn-Genet Recitas's "The Plan" diet, profiled in *More* magazine, http://more.com/weight-loss-diet-recitas.

[4]See Jamie Oliver, *Jamie's Food Revolution* (New York: Hyperion, 2009), and Alice Waters, *The Art of Simple Food* (New York: Clarkson Potter, 2007).

[5]See especially Michael Pollan, *In Defense of Food* (New York: Penguin, 2009); Mark Bittman, *Food Matters Cookbook* (New York: Simon & Schuster, 2010); and Barbara Kingsolver with Stephen Hopp and Camille Kingsolver, *Animal, Vegetable, Miracle* (New York: Harper Perennial, 2008).

[6]Both are still excellent resources that are well worth a look.

[7]The Slow Food movement was started by Carlo Petrini, an Italian who was dismayed by McDonald's presence in some of Rome's most historic piazzas. His book *Slow Food Nation: Why Our Food Should Be Clean, Good, and Fair* (New York: Rizzoli Ex Libris, 2007) is well worth a read.

[8]Victor Hugo, *Les Miserables, a Novel,* trans. Charles Edwin Wilbur (New York: Carleton Publishers, 1863), p. 8. See also Caroline Walker Bynum's seminal work *Holy Feast and Holy Fast: The Religious Significance of Food to Medieval Women,* The New Historicism: Studies in Cultural Poetics (Berkeley: University of California Press, 1988).

Chapter 1: Joyful Eating

[1]Psalm 104 is significant in this regard: God feeds all.

[2]A Jewish school focusing on the study of religious texts, including the Torah and the Talmud.

[3]Lisa Velthouse, *Craving Grace* (Carol Stream, IL: Tyndale House, 2011), p. 18.

[4]Phyllis Trible, *God and the Rhetoric of Sexuality* (Philadelphia: Fortress Press, 1978), p. 18.

[5]See Albert Y. Hsu's thoughts on theologian Robert Webber's insights on eating and fellowship in *Singles at the Crossroads: A Fresh Perspective on Christian Singleness* (Downers Grove, IL: InterVarsity Press, 1997), p. 132.

[6]Judi Barrett and Ron Barrett (illustrator), *Cloudy with a Chance of Meat-*

balls (New York: Simon & Schuster, 1978). It's worth reading the book; it's far superior to the film adaptation!

[7] "Eyeful of breast-feeding mom sparks outrage," Associated Press July 27, 2006, http://msnbc.msn.com/id/14065706/ns/health-womens _health.

[8] I made a similar case defending a silly breastfeeding doll from indecency charges in my brief article "What's the Big Deal About Baby Gloton?" https://catapultmagazine.com/babies-everywhere/review/whats-the-big-deal-about-bebe-gloton, and again on the *Christianity Today* women's blog, when a woman claimed she'd been thrown out of church for breast-feeding: http://blog.christianitytoday.com/women/2012/03/the_best_ place_to_breastfeed_i.html.

[9] When a baby nurses, the mother's body secretes oxytocin, a neurotrans-mitter nicknamed the "love hormone," understood to be responsible for promoting feelings of caring, trust, closeness and generosity.

[10] No, I'm not a "boob Nazi." Formula is invaluable in many situations—as in situations involving breast deformity, adoptions, HIV/AIDS and others—but there are good reasons to advocate for breastfeeding when possible, not least because it is the safest, healthiest, most affordable option for women in the developing world. See my post at http://eatwithjoy.org/2011/08/08/breastfeeding-and-justice/.

[11] I'm aware that complicated relationships with earthly mothers who were and/or are less than unconditionally loving may complicate this met-aphor for some people, just as imagining God as Father is troublesome for people who don't share a good relationship with their own fathers. What is in mind, however, is an ideal, unconditional-love relationship.

[12] The Hebrew word for compassion is related to the Hebrew word for womb, suggesting that compassion is kind of a "womb-ache," an ex-tension of motherly tenderness. Some Hebrew scholars dislike this reading, though. Again see Phyllis Trible, *God and the Rhetoric of Sexu-ality* (Philadelphia: Fortress Press, 1978), p. 33.

[13] Wendell Berry, "The Pleasures of Eating." Full text online at http://ecoliteracy.org/essays/pleasures-eating and in Norman Wirzba, ed., *The Art of the Commonplace: The Agrarian Essays of Wendell Berry* (Berkeley, Calif.: Counterpoint, 2002).

[14] I am using the word *sacramental* here in the sense of "an outward and physical sign of an inward and spiritual grace." There is debate over whether or not Jesus is in fact establishing the celebration of the Lord's Supper in John 6, and I'm not entering into it, just suggesting that we might reasonably consider all our eating to be an outward, physical sign of our inward, spiritual dependence on Christ.

[15]See my conversation with Norman Wirzba at the *Christianity Today* women's blog at http://blog.christianitytoday.com/women/2011/09/inviting _christ_to_the_dinner.html.

[16]It's worth noting that the very next verses of that psalm feature a food/wisdom motif:

> Faithfulness will spring up from the ground,
>   and righteousness will look down from the sky.
> The Lord will give what is good,
>   and our land will yield its increase. (Ps. 85:11-12)

[17]"Babette's Feast," *Anecdotes of Destiny and Ehrengard* (New York: Vintage International Paperbacks, 1993). That Isak Dinesen (aka Karen Blixen) may have died from anorexia is a sadly ironic background to the masterful tale and beautiful film.

[18]Ellyn Satter, *Secrets of Feeding a Healthy Family* (Madison, WI: Kelcy Press, 1999), p. 13, emphasis original.

[19]Sydney Spiesel, "The Skinny on Kids' Diets," *Slate*, December 19, 2006, http://slate.com/articles/health_and_science/medical_examiner/2006/12/the_skinny_on_kids_diets.html. See also C. M. Davis, "Results of the Self-selection of Diets by Young Children," *Canadian Medical Association Journal* 41 (1939): 257-61.

[20]Satter, *Secrets of Feeding a Healthy Family*, p. 7.

[21]Richard Bauckham, *The Bible and Ecology* (Waco, TX: Baylor University Press, 2010), p. 73.

[22]"Commentary on Acts 16:25-34: Dangerous Joy," *Third Way Magazine*, September 2006, p. 20.

[23]Anne Lamott, *Bird by Bird: Some Instructions on Writing and Life* (New York: Anchor Books, 1994), p. 179.

[24]See C. S. Lewis's brilliant and brief essay "First and Second Things" in *God in the Dock* (Grand Rapids: Eerdmans, 1970).

[25]Michael Pollan, *The Omnivore's Dilemma* (New York: Penguin, 2006), p. 3; P. Rozin, C. Fischler, S. Imada, A. Sarubin and A. Wzesmiewski, "Attitudes to Food and the Role of Food in Life in the U.S.A., Japan, Flemish Belgium and France: Possible Implications for the Diet-Health Debate," *Appetite* 33, no. 2 (October 1999): 163-80.

Chapter 2: Generous Eating

[1]Stephen H. Webb, *Good Eating* (Grand Rapids: Brazos, 2001).

[2]*Deus Caritas Est* §22.

[3]Kevin DeYoung and Greg Gilbert, *What Is the Mission of the Church?* (Wheaton, IL: Crossway Books, 2011). See my full critique in *Relevant*

at http://relevantmagazine.com/culture/books/reviews/27314-review
-what-is-the-mission-of-the-church.

[4]Christopher Hays, "Provision for the Poor and the Mission of the
Church: Ancient Appeals and Contemporary Viability," presented at
the 2011 Prestige FOCUS Conference on Mission and Ethics at the University of Pretoria, South Africa. Chris is a British Academy Postdoc-
toral Fellow with a PhD in New Testament wealth ethics who plans to
spend his career teaching in the Majority World.

[5]Marilynne Robinson, "The Fate of Ideas: Moses," in *When I Was a Child
I Read Books* (New York: Farrar, Straus & Giroux, 2012).

[6]Augustus Gloop was Roald Dahl's greedy character in *Charlie and the
Chocolate Factory*, whose girth stopped up a chocolate pipeline in the
Wonka factory.

[7]Pam Belluck, "Obesity Rates Hit Plateau in U.S., Data Suggest," *New
York Times,* January 13, 2010.

[8]Noted everywhere; one of my favorite books mentioning this is Michael Pollan's *In Defense of Food* (New York: Penguin, 2010), p. 112.

[9]Eric Jaffe, "Word to Your Mother," http://psychologicalscience.org/
index.php/publications/observer/2010/july-august-10/word-to-your-
mother.html.

[10]Simon Langley-Evans, *Nutrition: A Lifespan Approach* (Ames, IA: Wiley-
Blackwell, 2009), p. 66.

[11]See, for example, Michele Simon's *Appetite for Profit: How the Food Industry Undermines Our Health and How to Fight Back* (New York: Nation
Books, 2006).

[12]For example, see Mary Story and Simone French, "Food Advertising
and Marketing Directed at Children and Adolescents in the United
States," *International Journal of Behavioral Nutrition and Physical Activity* 1 (2004): 3.

[13]Kelly Brownell, *Food Fight: The Inside Story of the Food Industry, America's Obesity Crisis, and What We Can Do About It* (New York: McGraw-
Hill, 2004).

[14]This is part of the reason many of us struggle with our weight—the
food we're eating is addictive and calorically dense *by design.* Kessler's
book *The End of Overeating* (New York: Rodale, 2009) is worth reading.
He talks at length about how the industry capitalizes on these taste
preferences to create "hyper-palatable" foods that are all but impossible not to overeat and become addicted to.

[15]N. D. Volkow et al., "'Nonhedonic' Food Motivation in Humans Involves Dopamine in the Dorsal Striatum, and Methylphenidate Am-
plifies This Effect," *Synapse* 44, no. 3 (June 2002): 175-80.

[16]A. Drewnowski, M. Maillot and N. Darmon, "Testing Nutrient Profile Models in Relation to Energy Density and Energy Cost," *European Journal of Clinical Nutrition* (February 20, 2008).

[17]A. Drewnowski and S. E. Specter, "Poverty and Obesity: The Role of Energy Density and Energy Costs," *American Journal of Clinical Nutrition* 79, no. 1 (January 2004): 6-16.

[18]John Cawley and Chad Meyerhoefer, "The Medical Care Costs of Obesity," *National Bureau of Economic Research Working Paper No. 16467* (October 2010).

[19]Not his real name.

[20]Staffan Lindeberg, *Food and Western Disease: Health and Nutrition from an Evolutionary Perspective* (Ames, IA: Wiley-Blackwell, 2010). During a month-long visit with a friend in Paris, I could not help but notice the large amounts of packaged junk food even in Parisian supermarkets. Rates of obesity and diet-related disease, in France as everywhere, are on the rise.

[21]Peter Menzel and Faith D'Aluzio, *Hungry Planet: What the World Eats* (Napa, CA: Material World, 2005).

[22]Some think Jesus is the name of a French priest. See "Coca-Cola is more popular than Jesus," http://withinreachglobal.org/field-blog/dj/01-16-11/coca-cola-more-popular-jesus.

[23]Many books have convinced me that this is the case, but two of them stand out in connection with this. The first is Brian Wansink's *Mindless Eating: Why We Eat More Than We Think* (New York: Bantam, 2010). Wansink is a researcher who directs the Cornell Food and Brand Lab at Cornell University. Through numerous quirky and fascinating studies, he has demonstrated how things like portion size, color, variety and plate size influence people to eat more than they think they're eating. Kelly Brownell, Yale professor and director of Yale's Rudd Center for Food Policy and Obesity, has argued in his book *Food Fight,* coauthored with Katherine Battle Horgen (Chicago: Contemporary Books, 2004), and elsewhere that America's "toxic food environment"— shaped by the food industry in accordance with and capitalizing on the same kinds of tendencies that Wansink notes and the same inborn taste preferences that scientists agree we have—is guilty of recklessly endangering national health.

[24]Michael Pollan, *The Omnivore's Dilemma* (New York: Penguin Books, 2006).

[25]I'm in agreement with the majority of film reviewers evaluating *Fast Food Nation* as a lame adaptation of an awesome book by Eric Schlosser (New York: Harper Perennial, 2005). Nonetheless, while I urge people

to read Schlosser's book, I also realize that people are busy, and watching a 1 hour 45 minute movie is a lot more realistic for most people than reading a 400-page, research-heavy book. Additionally, I think the shocking and disturbing visual images do a lot to impress our imaginations with at least an inkling of the reality they represent.

[26]*Blood, Sweat, and Fear,* Human Rights Watch (2005), www.hrw.org/en/reports/2005/01/24/blood-sweat-and-fear.

[27]Upton Sinclair, *The Jungle* (numerous editions available). If your child reads it in school, urge them and their teacher to reflect as well on the current situation of meatpacking workers.

[28]The short PBS American Experience documentary titled *The Triangle Fire* demonstrates how the Triangle tragedy gripped the nation viscerally and led directly to the passage of federal employment laws and increased workers' rights. In the interest of letting you know where I'm coming from, my foremothers (on all sides of my heritage: Irish, French-Canadian and Eastern European Jewish) worked at factory jobs just like the Triangle shirtwaist girls. I suppose that inevitably their stories and legacy—combined with my conviction that God has a deep love and concern for poor immigrants—have shaped my awareness and concern for workers' rights.

[29]Human Rights Watch's *Blood, Sweat, and Fear* echoes Eric Schlosser's excellent reporting in *Fast Food Nation.*

[30]*Blood, Sweat, and Fear,* p. 46.

[31]Ibid., p. 52.

[32]Cynthia Kadohata, *Kira-Kira* (New York: Simon & Schuster, 2004). The Newbery Medal is given annually to the author of the most distinguished contribution to American literature for children. Like many Newbery novels, *Kira-Kira* is a compelling read for all ages. You can watch a documentary, *20,000 Cuts a Day,* produced by PBS's Expose series that tells stories much like *Kira Kira,* http://pbs.org/wnet/expose/2008/06/304-index.html.

[33]See http://companypay.com/executive/compensation/tyson-foods-inc.asp?yr=2007.

[34]Tracie McMillan, *The American Way of Eating* (New York: Scribner, 2012), p. 29.

[35]Susie Shellenberger, *Secret Power to Faith, Family and Getting a Guy* (Grand Rapids: Zondervan, 2006); Jackie Kendall and Debbie Jones, *Lady in Waiting: Becoming God's Best While Waiting for Mr. Right* (Shippensburg, PA: Destiny Image Publishers, 1995).

[36]I'm very much indebted to my husband, Timothy J. Stone, and the excellent research and insight summarized in his paper "Six Measures of

Barley," presented at the 2010 meeting of the Society of Biblical Literature in Atlanta.

[37]Marilynne Robinson, "Open Thy Hand Wide," in *When I Was A Child I Read Books*, p. 77.

[38]The more respectful term is undocumented worker. I'm trying to highlight that Boaz was under legal requirement to exclude Ruth, but he nonetheless included her as intimately as one could.

[39]Bread for the World runs a blog (http://blog.bread.org) that's a great resource for keeping current with hunger politics worldwide. You can also sign up for an account with Change.org, where you can either create petitions or keep informed on petitions created by others in requesting fair wages for agricultural workers, responsible business practices and other significant issues.

[40]See www.huffingtonpost.com/shane-claiborne/practicing-resurrection-t_b_1443621.html?ref=food&ir=Food.

[41]Wendell Berry, "Mad Farmer Liberation Front," from *The Country of Marriage* (New York: Harcourt Brace Jovanovich, 1973).

[42]Sara Miles's book *Take This Bread* (New York: Ballantine Books, 2008) is in part about her church's effort to do just this.

[43]I'm aware of Coca-Cola's "clean water" initiative. However, I think my point still stands. While I'll enjoy a soda every now and then, I still feel that the amount of energy and water consumed in the production of the "liquid candy" that is Coke is unjustifiably wasteful when so many still lack reliable access to clean drinking water.

[44]Janet Morley, "Christian Aid," *Harvest for the World: A Worship Anthology on Sharing in the Work of Creation* (Cleveland: Pilgrim Press, 2003), p. 149.

[45]Huron Hunger Fund, Anglican Church of Canada, in *Blessed Be Our Table*, ed. Neil Paynter (Glasgow: Wild Goos Publications, 2003).

[46]Nicaraguan Prayer and Armenian Prayer found in *Blessed Be Our Table*.

Chapter 3: Communal Eating

[1]Richard Wrangham, *Catching Fire: How Cooking Made Us Human* (New York: Basic Books, 2010).

[2]Diane Ackerman, "The Social Sense," in *Food and Faith*, ed. Michael Schut (New York: Morehouse Publishing, 2002).

[3]Abraham Rosman, Paula G. Rubel and Maxine Weisgrau, *The Tapestry of Culture: An Introduction to Cultural Anthropology*, 9th ed. (Lanham, MD: Altamira Press, 2009), p. 8.

[4]See Craig Blomberg's *Contagious Holiness: Jesus' Meals with Sinners*, New Studies in Biblical Theology (Downers Grove, IL: IVP Academic, 2005).

196

EAT WITH JOY

[5]David Seccombe, quoted in Blomberg, *Contagious Holiness*, p. 19.

[6]Quoted in Marilynne Robinson, *When I Was a Child I Read Books* (New York: Farrar, Straus & Giroux, 2012), pp. 82-83.

[7]Philip Yancey, *What's So Amazing About Grace?* (Grand Rapids: Zondervan, 2002), p. 148.

[8]Christine D. Pohl, *Making Room* (Grand Rapids: Eerdmans, 1999), pp. 5, 32.

[9]Ibid., p. 36.

[10]Ibid., p. 74.

[11]"Portrait of the Meal-for-One Society," January 30, 2004, http://news.bbc.co.uk/2/hi/uk_news/magazine/3445091.stm.

[12]ChildTrendsDatabase.org, "The More We Eat Together: State Data on Frequency of Family Meals."

[13]Edith Schaeffer, *The Tapestry* (Waco, TX: Word Books, 1984).

[14]Nora Ephron, in *The Family Dinner* by Laurie David with Kirstin Uhrenholdt (New York: Grand Central Life & Style, 2010).

[15]Pohl, *Making Room*, p. 73.

[16]Jodi Kantor, *The Obamas* (New York: Hachette Books, 2012).

[17]Robert Farrar Capon, *Between Noon and Three: Romance, Law, and the Outrage of Grace* (Grand Rapids: Eerdmans, 1997).

Chapter 4: Restorative Eating

[1]Lauren Greenfield, *Thin* (San Francisco: Chronicle Books, 2006), introduction by Joan Jacobs Brumberg.

[2]Ibid., p. 71.

[3]Ibid., pp. 81, 83.

[4]Ibid., p. 40.

[5]Ibid., p. 48.

[6]Shelly Guillory, "Shelly Speaks," http://mamavision.com/2009/08/08/shelly-from-thin-documentary-five-years-later/.

[7]"Polly Williams of HBOs Thin Found Dead," www.accesshollywood.com/Polly-Williams-Of-HBOs-Thin-Found-Dead_article_8390.

[8]I am grateful for the opportunity to exchange email with Shelly Guillory. Thank you, Shelly! Though I did not receive replies from other women in *Thin* whom I contacted, I want to honor them and wish them continued healing.

[9]Hilda Bruch, *The Golden Cage: The Enigma of Anorexia Nervosa* (Cambridge, MA: Harvard University Press, 2001).

[10]Harriet Brown writes about Ancel Keys's experiment in *Brave Girl Eating: A Family's Struggle with Anorexia* (New York: William Morrow, 2010); Lynne Gerber, in *Seeking the Straight and Narrow: Weight Loss*

and *Sexual Reorientation in Evangelical America* (Chicago: University of Chicago Press, 2012). A good summary is available in *Journal of Nutrition* 135, no. 6 (June 1, 2005): 1347-52; online at http://jn.nutrition .org/content/135/6/1347.full.

[11]Brown, *Brave Girl Eating*, p. 83.

[12]Laura Collins, *Eating with Your Anorexic: How My Child Recovered Through Family-Based Treatment and Yours Can Too* (New York: McGraw-Hill, 2005), p. 160.

[13]Brown, *Brave Girl Eating*, p. 71.

[14]Gerard Manley Hopkins, "The Kingfisher": "The just man justices / Keeps grace: that keeps all his goings graces." www.poetryfoundation .org/poem/173654 (in the public domain).

[15]Eric Stice at http://time.com/time/nation/article/0,8599,2025345,00 .html#ixzz1ByKJIYWO.

[16]Anne Lamott, *Bird by Bird* (New York: Anchor Books, 2004), p. 170.

[17]See www.people.com/people/archive/article/0,,20150380,00.html.

Chapter 5: Sustainable Eating

[1]We visited the unimaginatively named yet beautiful lakes known as Arch Lake, Little Arch Lake and Upper Arch Lake.

[2]Gerard Manley Hopkins, "God's Grandeur" (1877; in the public domain).

[3]Nancy Pearcey and Charles B. Thaxton, *The Soul of Science: Christian Faith and Natural Philosophy* (Wheaton, IL: Crossway Books, 1994), p. 35. Pearcey insists that naming, in Hebrew, implies mastery. In *The Bible and Ecology: Rediscovering the Community of Creation* (Waco, TX: Baylor University Press, 2010), Richard Bauckham cites this frequent assumption, saying that "there is no good reason" to understand the Hebrew in this way.

[4]Preface to *Making Peace with the Land* by Fred Bahnson and Norman Wirzba (Downers Grove, IL: InterVarsity Press, 2012).

[5]Marilynne Robinson, "The Human Spirit and the Good Society," in *When I Was a Child I Read Books* (New York: Farrar, Strauss & Giroux, 2012), p. 162.

[6]Marilynne Robinson, "The Fate of Ideas: Moses," in *When I Was a Child I Read Books,* p. 106.

[7]United Methodist Hymnal no. 227, www.hymnary.org/hymn/UMH/227.

[8]I especially love Sufjan Stevens's recording of this song on his *Songs for Christmas* album.

[9]Thomas of Celano, *First Life of Saint Francis,* nos. 58-60, 80-81.

[10]Psalm 8 balances humans as lower than angels but higher than animals.

[11]Bauckham, *Bible and Ecology,* pp. 145, 147.

[12]Bill McKibben, *The Comforting Whirlwind* (New York: Cowley Publications, 2005). See also his *The End of Nature* (New York: Random House, 2006).

[13]Bauckham calls Job 38–39 "strong medicine" against human arrogance, in *Bible and Ecology,* p. 37.

[14]Daniel Block, in *Keeping God's Earth,* ed. Daniel Block & Noah J. Toly (Downers Grove, IL: InterVarsity Press, 2010), pp. 126-32.

[15]Robinson, *When I Was a Child I Read Books.*

[16]Bauckham, in *Bible and Ecology,* p. 175.

[17]Richard Stearns, *The Hole in Our Gospel* (Nashville: Thomas Nelson, 2009), p. 69.

[18]Michael Pollan, "Farmer in Chief," *New York Times,* October 10, 2009.

[19]Carolyn Dimitri, Anne Effland and Neilson Conklin, "Environmental Protection Agency Agriculture 101 fact sheet—Demographics," http://epa.gov/oecaagct/ag101/demographics.html, and "The 20th Century Transformation of U.S. Agriculture and Farm Policy," Electronic Information Bulletin Number 3, June 2005, http://ers.usda.gov/publications/eib3/eib3.htm.

[20]R. Das, A. Steege, S. Baron, J. Beckman and R. Harrison, "Pesticide-Related Illness Among Migrant Farm Workers in the United States," *International Journal of Occupational and Environmental Health* 7, no. 4 (October-December 2001): 303-12; P. K. Mills and R. C. Yang, "Agricultural Exposures and Gastric Cancer Risk in Hispanic Farm Workers in California," in *Environmental Resesearch* 104, no. 2 (June 2007): 282-89; Occupational Health Branch, California Department of Health Services, Oakland, USA.

[21]Michael Pollan, "What's Eating America?" *Smithsonian* (June 15, 2006), available at www.michaelpollan.com; also see the biography of Haber at Chemical Heritage Foundation website: http://chemheritage.org/discover/chemistry-in-history/themes/early-chemistry-and-gases/haber.aspx.

[22]See http://ers.usda.gov/Data/BiotechCrops/ExtentofAdoptionTable1.htm.

[23]*The Future of Food,* directed by Deborah Koons Garcia (2004).

[24]Gregory Johanssen, "When Genetically Modified Crops Go Wild," http://environmentalgraffiti.com/plants/news-first-genetically-modified-crop-found-wild.

[25]Greenpeace,"Golden Rice: All Glitter, No Gold" (March 16, 2005), http://greenpeace.org/international/en/news/features/failures-of-golden-rice, and "Golden Rice a Distraction to Solving Vitamin A Deficiency" (November 9, 2010), www.greenpeace.org/seasia/news/Golden-

Rice-a-distraction-to-solving-Vitamin-A-deficiency.

[26]"Monsanto Donates Corn and Vegetable Seeds to Haiti," Monsanto.com (2010); Beverly Bell, "Haitian Farmers Commit to Burning Monsanto Hybrid Seeds," May 18, 2010, www.truth-out.org/haitian-farmers-commit-burning-monsanto-hybrid-seeds59616.

[27]Christos Vasilikiotis, "Can Organic Farming 'Feed the World'?" www.cnr.berkeley.edu/~christos/articles/cv_organic_farming.html.

[28]The claim is that labeling GM crops may create unnecessary fears, e.g., C. A. Carter and G. P. Gruere, "Mandatory Labeling of Genetically Modified Foods: Does It Really Provide Consumer Choice?" *AgBio Forum* 6, no. 18 (2003): www.agbioforum.org/.

[29]A wide-ranging overview of the pros and cons of genetically modified foods appears at www.csa.com/discoveryguides/gmfood/overview.php.

[30]Eric Schlosser, *Fast Food Nation* (New York: Houghton Mifflin, 2001).

[31]Documentary film *Future of Food*.

[32]Ken Midkiff, *The Meat You Eat: How Corporate Farming Has Endangered America's Food Supply* (New York: St. Martin's Griffin, 2005), p. 2.

[33]Michael Pollan makes this point in his follow-up to *The Omnivore's Dilemma*, the powerful *In Defense of Food*: "Your health isn't bordered by your body, and what's good for the soil is probably good for you, too" (New York: Penguin, 2009), p. 169.

[34]John H. Vandermeer, *The Ecology of Agroecosystems* (Sudbury, MA: Jones and Bartlett, 2011), pp. 4-8.

[35]Block, *Keeping God's Earth*, p. 116.

[36]Ibid., p. 122.

[37]"Saving Species," *Planet Earth: The Future*, produced by Fergus Beeley (2006).

[38]"Planting Trees of Peace," www.greenbeltmovement.org/a.php?id=90.

[39]Barbara Kingsolver, with Steven Hopp and Camille Kingsolver, *Animal, Vegetable, Miracle* (New York: Harper Perennial, 2008), pp. 54-57.

[40]I have found William Webb's "redemptive-movement" hermeneutic very helpful in navigating the tricky world of biblical interpretation and application. His book *Slaves, Women and Homosexuals* (Downers Grove, IL: IVP Academic, 2001) and his contribution to *Moving Beyond the Bible to Theology* explain this concept, which holds that divine prescriptions within Scripture cannot always be understood as representative of God's ideals for all people at all times; rather, they represent his work with specific people in specific contexts. For example, the epistle's instructions to "greet one another with a holy kiss," applied literally, would make many men in North America feel very uncomfortable—which is opposite the intention behind that instruction.

[41]Stephen H. Webb, *Good Eating* (Grand Rapids: Brazos, 2001), p. 226.

[42]John Robbins's classic *Diet for a New America* (Novato, CA: New World Library, 1987) is worth a look; so is the more current *Eating Animals* by Jonathan Safran Foer (New York: Little, Brown & Company, 2009).

[43]Kendra Langdon Juskus, "A Call to Compassion from Our Brothers the Animals," *Prism* (July/August 2011), pp. 19-22.

[44]Bauckham, *Bible and Ecology*, p. 136.

[45]Block, *Keeping God's Earth*, p. 135.

[46]Bauckham's translation, *Bible and Ecology*, p. 138.

[47]Block, *Keeping God's Earth*, p. 137.

[48]Ibid., p. 139.

[49]Wendell Berry, *The Gift of Good Land* (New York: North Point Press, 1982), p. 279.

[50]Adapted from Mark Bittman's *Food Matters Cookbook* (New York: Simon & Schuster, 2010).

[51]Inspired by Elise Bauer's recipe on her excellent blog, *Simply Recipes*.

Chapter 6: Creative Eating

[1]Jean Anthelme Brillat-Savarin, *The Physiology of Taste: Or Meditations on Transcendental Gastronomy*, trans. M. F. K. Fisher (Washington, DC: Counterpoint, 1949), p. 158.

[2]Amy Tan, *The Joy Luck Club* (New York: Penguin Books, 1996), p. 178.

[3]John S. Allen, *The Omnivorous Mind: Our Evolving Relationship with Food* (Cambridge, MA: Harvard University Press, 2012), p. 3.

[4]Harvey Levenstein, *Paradox of Plenty: A Social History of Eating in Modern America*, California Studies in Food and Culture (Berkeley: University of California Press, 2003), p. 116.

[5]Lysa TerKeurst, *Made to Crave: Satisfying Your Deepest Desires with God, Not Food* (Grand Rapids: Zondervan, 2010).

[6]Andrew F. Smith, *Eating History: Thirty Turning Points in the Making of American Cuisine* (New York: Columbia University Press, 2009), p. 32.

[7]Francis Sizer and Ellie Whitney, *Nutrition: Concepts and Controversies*, 11th ed. (Belmont, CA: Thomson, 2008), p. 13.

[8]Robert Farrar Capon, *Supper of the Lamb: A Culinary Reflection* (New York: Modern Library, 2002), p. 20.

[9]Ibid., p. 21.

[10]I'm grateful to have had the opportunity to interview chefs Hayden and Fleming of the North Fork Table and Inn on the occasion of their being awarded a rare 29/30 for food on the Zagat survey. A small portion of our conversation appeared in our local paper, *The Suffolk Times*, May 20, 2011.

[11]Capon, *Supper of the Lamb*, p. 19.

[12]Ibid., p. 4.

[13]Dorothy Sayers, *The Mind of the Maker* (New York: Continuum, 2005), p. 129.

[14]"Ask yourself how many of these [convenience foods that wreck a sense of 'home'] declinations from the act of creation you allow in your vice-gerency. . . . Burger King has no throne for you to pretend to" (Robert Farrar Capon, *Capon on Cooking* [Boston: Houghton Mifflin, 1983]).

[15]See, for example, Mihaly Csikszentmihalyi, *Creativity: Flow and the Psychology of Discovery and Invention* (New York: HarperCollins, 1996).

[16]The PBS documentary *The Persuaders* explains how this tendency to make associations—even, and perhaps especially, irrational ones—promotes cravings and product sales. Directed by Barak Goodman and Rachel Dretzin, aired Nov. 9, 2003. WGBH Educational Foundation.

[17]Barbara Kingsolver, with Steven L. Hopp and Camille Kingsolver, *Animal, Vegetable, Miracle* (New York: HarperCollins, 2007), pp. 31-32.

[18]Kingsolver, radio interview with Krista Tippett, "The Ethics of Eating," American Public Radio's *Speaking of Faith/On Being*, July 15, 2010.

[19]G. K. Chesterton, *Orthodoxy* (Chicago: Moody Publishers, 2009), p. 64.

[20]Julia Child, *Julia's Kitchen Wisdom: Essential Techniques and Recipes from a Lifetime of Cooking* (New York: Borzoi Books, 2000), p. 3.

[21]Capon, *Capon on Cooking*, p. 172.

[22]Capon, *Supper of the Lamb*, p. 40.

Chapter 7: Redemptive Eating

[1]Marion Nestle, quoted in Michael Pollan, *In Defense of Food: An Eater's Manifesto* (New York: Penguin, 2008), p. 62.

[2]Malcolm Gladwell, "The Roseto Mystery," in *Outliers: The Story of Success* (New York: Little, Brown & Company, 2008), pp. 3-11.

[3]See our interview: "Inviting Christ to the Dinner Table," *Her.meneutics* blog, blog.christianitytoday.com/women/2011/09/inviting_Christ_to_the_dinner.html.

[4]Lynne Gerber, *Seeking the Straight and Narrow: Weight Loss and Sexual Reorientation in Evangelical America* (Chicago: University of Chicago Press, 2012), p. 141.

[5]Wendell Berry, "Think Little," in *The Art of the Commonplace: The Agrarian Essays of Wendell Berry,* ed. Norman Wirzba (Berkeley, CA: Counterpoint, 2002), p. 88.

[6]See Margaret Kim Peterson, *Keeping House: The Litany of Everyday Life* (San Francisco: Jossey-Bass, 2007), p. 110.

[7]See J. Brent Bill and Beth Booram, *Awaken Your Senses* (Downers Grove,

IL: IVP Books, 2012), pp. 22-57, for more mindfulness activities centered on experiencing the wonder of God and God's creation through the five senses.

[8]Thanks to Norman Wirzba, who articulated this idea beautifully in an interview with me for the *Christianity Today* women's blog *Her.meneutics*.

[9]William J. Webb, *Slaves, Women and Homosexuals* (Downers Grove, IL: IVP Academic, 2001).

[10]Doris Janzen Longacre, *More-with-Less* (Newton, KS: Herald Press, 1976), p. 23.

[11]Transcribed from N. T. Wright, "God's Light in the Post-Post Enlightenment World," *Christian Hope in a Postmodern World* (Vancouver, BC: Regent Audio, 2002), disc 3. This also appears almost word for word in Wright's book *The Challenge of Jesus* (Downers Grove, IL: InterVarsity Press, 1999), p. 188.

Name and Subject Index

addictive food, 48, 49, 194

agriculture, 14, 21, 60, 67, 113-18, 123, 124, 133, 142, 145, 164, 178

American Way of Eating, 56

anorexia, 15, 89, 93, 94, 95, 96, 99, 178, 193, 198

animals, 16, 24, 53, 54, 56, 108-12, 116, 118, 119-25

appetite, 38, 99, 135, 168

asceticism, 33, 89, 135-37, 139

Babette's Feast, 33-35, 181, 193

Bauckham, Richard, 110, 121, 193

Berry, Wendell, 31, 32, 125, 163, 178, 179

Bible, 18, 29, 30, 57, 58, 59, 108, 109, 110, 112, 118, 120, 121, 136, 137, 148, 170, 193, 199

biodiversity, 118-19, 125, 184

Bittman, Mark, 16, 41, 179

body image, 13, 14, 18, 46, 89-93, 97, 104

Bread for the World, 61, 130, 197

bread of life, 20, 22, 35, 37, 39, 40, 44, 59

breastfeeding, 28, 47, 192

breasts, 28-29, 180

bulimia, 89

calories, 9, 38, 48, 49, 67, 91, 96, 101, 124, 138, 139, 140, 184

Candy Land, 90

Capon, Robert F., 82, 136, 138-40, 142, 150, 151, 177, 178

celebration, 32, 139, 160, 165, 166, 167, 175, 192

Child, Julia, 146, 149, 150, 151, 157, 203

childhood obesity, 15

children, 11, 14, 15, 16, 17, 36-37, 46, 47, 48, 62, 71, 75-76, 78, 80, 104, 147, 161

Christian diets, 13-14, 18, 91, 137, 157, 161

church, 13, 17, 18, 33, 34, 44, 53, 62, 65, 67, 68-70, 75, 77, 79, 82, 91, 100, 109, 135, 166, 168, 172, 175, 181, 182, 184, 194

Claiborne, Shane, 61, 197

Coca-Cola, 17, 52, 195, 197

communion, 19, 25, 112

Communion, 24, 32, 33, 42, 68, 77, 100, 160

community, 22, 25, 45, 61, 64, 66, 75, 79, 92, 98, 108, 110, 159, 167, 173, 181
    of creation, 108, 110, 199

company, 35, 78, 79, 87, 101, 130, 166, 168

compassion, 29, 79, 121, 124

cooking, 13, 16, 19, 21-22, 26, 30, 62, 80, 97, 119, 134, 136, 138-42, 144, 146, 148-51

corn (industrial), 17, 49, 62, 113-19, 121-22, 162, 200

cost per calorie, 49

creation (natural world), 20, 21, 28, 37, 38, 72, 83, 107-13, 119, 120, 123, 125, 139, 141, 142, 145, 151, 156, 162, 165, 178, 183, 199

creativity, 62, 77, 134, 139, 141-43, 148, 150, 159-60, 165, 167

culinary arts, 24, 67, 72, 134, 167

desire, 9, 13, 23, 38, 94, 100, 104, 147, 152

diabetes, 46, 49, 52, 95, 137, 176

diet, 12, 13,16, 18, 36, 38, 39, 46, 49, 50, 52, 62, 75, 91, 97, 115, 118, 122, 123, 135, 136, 137, 139, 157, 158, 159, 166, 168

early church, 18, 33, 68, 181, 182

eating disorder, 12, 21, 22, 75, 78, 89, 92, 93, 95, 99, 101, 182, 183

eating together, 9, 21, 45, 67-68, 70-75, 77

Ehrenreich, Barbara, 51, 177

environment, 16, 52, 95, 107, 110, 112, 121, 200

Eucharist, 32, 33, 76

fair trade/fair food, 61, 63, 162, 164, 173

family, 12, 15, 23, 44, 46, 49, 56, 59, 70-72, 75-79, 82-83, 87, 88, 93-95

family meals, 72, 75, 78, 178, 182, 198
family-based therapy, 95-98
farm bill, 61
farm subsidies, 49, 50, 62, 162, 181
fast food, 17, 48-49, 61, 117, 162, 181
Fast Food Nation, 53, 182, 195, 196, 201
First Place, 161
food deserts, 51
Food, Inc., 49, 53, 184
food pantries, 15, 62
Francis of Assisi, St., 110
Free to Be Thin, 13, 14, 91
generosity, 37, 58, 59, 62, 65
genetically modified food (GMO), 113, 115-16, 200, 201
Gerber, Lynne, 13, 161
G.I. Joe, 90
giving thanks, 105, 151-52, 168, 185
gluten, 15, 75, 128, 129
gluttony, 38, 52
gospel, 43-45, 67, 68, 76, 169
grace, 9, 10, 19, 20, 33, 35, 60, 80-82, 83, 100, 101, 142, 151
gratitude, 38, 39, 65, 80, 148, 161, 163, 167-68
guilt, 12, 22, 38, 39, 52, 92, 94, 111, 161
Haber, Fritz, 113-14
healthy eating, 15, 39, 137
Heifer International, 124, 130
Human Rights Watch, 54, 196
hunger, 21, 23, 27, 29, 33, 37, 38, 44, 45, 51, 54, 63, 64, 65, 73, 74, 100, 136
hospitality, 9, 58, 69, 77, 82, 182
"hyperpalatability," 48
images of thinness, 90
industrial food, 9, 14, 16, 52, 114, 115, 146
Jesus, 9, 10, 11, 13, 18, 21, 22, 31-33, 34, 35, 37, 43-46, 52-53, 56, 59, 61, 62, 67, 68
joyful eating, 20, 21, 23, 145, 166-68, 170, 172, 180, 185
Jungle, The, 54, 196
justice, 19, 22, 46, 50, 53, 54, 56, 57-61, 63, 162, 172, 177
Kingsolver, Barbara, 16, 124, 145, 147, 178

Kira-Kira (novel), 56, 196
kosher, 69, 134
land, 17, 31, 59, 108, 109, 111, 113, 122, 125, 159, 178, 183, 193
law (biblical), 21, 45, 57-59, 62, 68, 109, 170
Lord's Supper, 10, 33, 42, 45, 77, 192
Maathai, Wangari, 118-19, 183
manna, 22, 27-31, 40
McDonald's, 21, 49, 117, 145, 162, 163, 176, 191
Morton Salt, 90
Mostly Martha, 72-74, 182
Nestle, Marion, 158, 159, 177, 185
Nobel Prize, 113, 118
nutrition, 37, 46, 61, 115, 135-37, 144, 151, 158, 175
Obama family, 76, 198
obesity, 15, 46, 47, 99, 194, 195
organic, 12, 15, 42, 51, 86, 112-13, 116, 128, 130, 137, 163, 164, 170, 201
OSHA, 55
overeating, 38, 48, 89, 101, 194
overweight, 47, 62, 91, 159
parents, 28, 29, 36, 47, 71, 104
and eating disorders, 94-95, 97
perfection, 13, 39, 80-81, 90, 91, 95, 135, 139, 168, 169, 170
pleasure, 16, 18, 24, 33, 36, 37, 38, 39, 40, 47, 78, 88, 94, 101, 107, 109, 134-38, 145, 151, 160, 167, 181, 184, 192
Pohl, Christine, 69, 70, 198
Pollan, Michael, 16, 39, 48, 113, 159, 169, 178
potato famine, 117-18
potluck, 74, 75, 79, 175, 182
poverty, 45, 49, 51, 56, 60, 119, 162, 195
Proverbs, 121
Psalms (biblical book), 35, 118, 152, 191, 193, 199
Renfrew Center, 92-95, 101, 183
restaurants, 23, 30, 35, 49, 66, 72, 73, 74, 80, 92, 131, 140, 142, 168
Robinson, Marilynne, 46, 108, 109, 111
Ruth (biblical), 21, 57-59, 62

Salatin, Joel, 53, 56, 122
Satter, Ellyn, 36-38, 161, 179, 193
sexuality, 14, 19, 24, 29, 46, 90, 136, 191, 192, 203
sharing, 9, 20, 21, 37, 45, 67, 69, 70, 76, 98, 133, 172, 175, 197
simplicity, 33, 65, 165, 166, 168, 175
Sinclair, Upton, 54, 196
slimming of toys, 90
Slow Food, 147, 168, 175, 191
slowness, 42, 147, 156, 160, 167-68, 171, 176
SNAP/food stamps, 15
starvation, 15, 27, 57, 94, 96
Strawberry Shortcake, 90
sugar, 15, 17, 46, 47, 48, 52, 162, 166, 169
sustainability, 21, 78, 106-128, 130, 170, 183, 199
table fellowship, 25, 67, 69, 75, 92, 181

veganism, vegan, 18, 69, 122, 124, 135, 137, 176
vegetarian(ism), 120-23, 135, 159, 167
wages, 15, 55, 56, 197
waste, 91, 126, 131
Webb, Stephen, 120, 193, 201
Webb, William, 170, 201
Weigh Down Diet, 13
weight, 11, 12, 14, 15, 16, 46, 47, 62, 91-93, 96, 101, 136, 161, 168
weight loss, 13, 14, 15, 16, 46, 92, 137, 168, 203
Weight Watchers, 13, 91, 139
White Rock girl, 90
Wirzba, Norman, 7, 10, 159, 177, 178, 192
wisdom, 25, 110, 168, 193
worker safety, 14, 54-56, 58, 62, 113, 196, 197, 200
World Vision, 44, 65, 130

Recipe Index

Beef and Beer Stew, 129
Black Bean and Corn Quinoa, 104
Bread, No-Knead, 41
Cinnamon Rolls, 153
Cucumber Salad, 64
Lentil Soup, Curried Red, 102
Lentil Soup, No Frills, 63
Orzo (Pasta) Summer Salad, 174

Peanut Sauce, 86
Peppermint Bark, 173
Potato Pancakes, 154
Ratatouille, 154
Spring/Summer Rolls, 85
Strawberry Rhubarb Pie, 84
Sweet Potato Fritters, 128

Scripture Index

OLD TESTAMENT

Genesis
1, 110, 120
1:28, 107
9, 120
9:1-3, 120
9:4, 121

Exodus
16:3, 27
23:9, 56
23:12, 121

Leviticus
23:22, 58
25:23, 109

Deuteronomy
5:14, 121
15, 68
15:11, 37
22:1-3, 121
23:3, 58
24:14, 56
24:19, 58
32:11-13, 30
32:18, 30

Ruth
1:6, 58
1:16, 57
2:8-9, 58
2:12, 59
4:15, 59

Job
40:3-5, 110

Psalms
85:11, 34
148:7-13, 110

Proverbs
12:10, 121
14:31, 56
22:16, 56
29:7, 60

Ecclesiastes
7, 170

Isaiah
11:6, 108
11:7, 111
49:15, 29
55:1-2, 18

55:2, 137
66:12, 29

Hosea
4:1-3, 122

Amos
8:4-6, 50

NEW TESTAMENT

Matthew
11:19, 10
18:3-4, 37
19, 37
25, 69
25:31-40,
    44

Mark
2:16, 68
10:23, 45

Luke
7:34, 10
14:13, 68

John
4:34, 83
6, 31
6:12, 126
6:51, 31
6:54-56, 31
6:68-69, 32

Acts
2:45, 45
2:46-47, 45
10, 68
10:34-35, 69

Romans
1:25, 108
8:22, 111

1 Corinthians
11, 68, 77

James
2:15-17, 44

Revelation
22, 123

About the Author

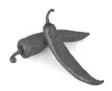

Rachel Marie Stone is a regular writer for *Christianity Today's* Her.meneutics blog. She has also written for such publications as *Christianity Today, Books & Culture, Catapult, Relevant, The Christian Century, Flourish* and *The Huffington Post.* She enjoys gardening and meal-making with her husband, an Old Testament scholar and professor at Zomba Theological College, Malawi, and two sons.

I would love to hear your stories of eating with joy, and, with your permission, to feature them on my blog (RachelMarieStone .com). Write to me at rachelmarie9@gmail.com.

Peace be with you!

LIKEWISE. *Go and do.*

A man comes across an ancient enemy, beaten and left for dead. He lifts the wounded man onto the back of a donkey and takes him to an inn to tend to the man's recovery. Jesus tells this story and instructs those who are listening to "go and do likewise."

Likewise books explore a compassionate, active faith lived out in real time. When we're skeptical about the status quo, Likewise books challenge us to create culture responsibly. When we're confused about who we are and what we're supposed to be doing, Likewise books help us listen for God's voice. When we're discouraged by the troubled world we've inherited, Likewise books encourage us to hold onto hope.

In this life we will face challenges that demand our response. Likewise books face those challenges with us so we can act on faith.

ivpress.com/likewise
twitter.com/likewise_books
facebook.com/likewisebooks
youtube.com/likewisebooks